FAST FACTS

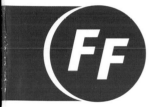

*Indispensable
Guides to
Clinical
Practice*

Dementia

To Many

best wishes

Lawrence

January 2003

Lawrence J Whalley

Professor of Mental Health,
University of Aberdeen Clinical Research Centre,
Royal Cornhill Hospital, Aberdeen, UK

John CS Breitner

Director, Geriatric Research Education and
Clinical Center, VA Puget Sound Health Care System,
Professor and Head, Division of Geriatric Psychiatry,
Department of Psychiatry and Behavioral Sciences,
University of Washington School of Medicine,
Seattle, Washington, USA

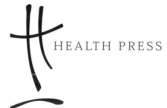

HEALTH PRESS

Oxford

Fast Facts – Dementia
First published November 2002

A CIP catalogue record for this title is available from the British
Library.

ISBN 1-899541-78-0

Whalley, LJ (Lawrence)
Fast Facts – Dementia/
Lawrence J Whalley, John CS Breitner

Medical illustrations by Dee McLean, London, UK.

Printed by Fine Print (Services) Ltd, Oxford, UK.

Glossary of abbreviations

ACh: acetylcholine

AChE: acetylcholinesterase

ACTH: adrenocorticotropic hormone

ADL: Activities of Daily Living

APP: amyloid precursor protein

CERAD: Consortium to Establish a Registry for Alzheimer's Disease

ChAT: choline acetyl transferase

DSM-IV: Diagnostic and Statistical Manual of Mental Disorders, 4th edition

DSRS: Dementia Symptom Rating Scale

DZ: dizygotic

GABA: gamma-amino butyric acid

ICD-10: International Statistical Classification of Diseases and Related Health Problems, 10th revision

MAP: microtubule-associated protein

MMSE: Mini Mental State Examination

MZ: monozygotic

NART: National Adult Reading Test

NFT: neurofibrillary tangle

NMDA: N-methyl-D-aspartate

NPI: Neuropsychiatric Inventory

NSAIDs: non-steroidal anti-inflammatory drugs

PET: positron emission tomography

PHFs: paired helical filaments

ROS: reactive oxygen species

SPECT: single photon emission computerized tomography

Introduction

It is almost 100 years since Alois Alzheimer first described the disease that bears his name, though the importance of his observations was not fully appreciated for almost 60 years. Until about 1970 medical undergraduates knew little about Alzheimer's disease, and most physicians attributed dementia in old age to hardening of the arteries of the brain and reserved the term 'Alzheimer's disease' for rare forms of presenile dementia. The last two decades have changed this. Now, more is known about the biology of Alzheimer's disease than about any other neuropsychiatric condition. Moreover, there is widespread public and professional awareness of dementia.

Dementia is not a single disorder, but a syndrome of mental life characterized by a global decline in cognitive ability that is not caused by an altered state of consciousness. It is most common in the elderly, in whom it usually results from Alzheimer's disease, cerebrovascular disease or both. Early symptoms typically reflect the type (presumed cause) of dementia and the parts of the brain most affected. Thereafter, with the progression of brain disease, usually all powers of memory and reasoning are eventually lost. Not all patients are aware of the change within them but those who are, not surprisingly, often experience important changes in outlook, including feelings of bleakness, powerlessness, or notions of dread, loathing or shame. Whether or not it is provoked by such feelings, or by the illness itself, the behavior of demented people often changes. Behavioral complications, such as irritability, resistance to offered help, wandering, 'rummaging' through closets or drawers, other 'automatic' behaviors such as picking at clothing or skin, are common and dramatically increase the burden of care.

Fast Facts – Dementia begins with a discussion of brain aging and its relationship to neurodegenerative disease, and then the cause, course and treatment of each of the common illnesses that can provoke the dementia syndrome are considered. Our aim is to enable the reader to understand the basic causes of dementia, recognize it clinically, appreciate the basic principles of investigation and management, and learn of some steps that may improve the long-term care of patients or perhaps even prevent dementia.

Because of its high prevalence and level of associated morbidity, dementia is already an urgent health and economic issue for the developed world. As public health efforts improve the life expectancy of populations in developing countries, the number of people with dementia worldwide is expected to quadruple by 2050. Effective means of intervention and prevention are thus needed urgently.

Basic science

Though the presence of dementia does not always imply the existence of an identifiable brain disease, it usually does so. A basic knowledge of some of the principles of neuroscience and the anatomy and physiology of the brain is therefore essential in beginning to understand the dementia syndrome.

Simple functional anatomy of the brain

An adult human brain weighs approximately 1.3 kg. The central nervous system of the adult brain is divided into six main parts: the spinal cord; the medulla, pons and midbrain that together comprise the brainstem; the diencephalon; and the cerebral hemispheres (Figure 1.1).

The largest components are the two cerebral hemispheres, which are principally responsible for the higher intellectual functions that distinguish humans from non-human primates. They consist of the cerebral cortex and three deep-lying structures:

- the basal ganglia, involved with regulation of motor performance
- the hippocampi, involved with memory
- the amygdaloid nuclei, involved with linkage of nervous and hormonal responses to emotions.

Deeper and older, in evolutionary terms, are the diencephalon and brainstem. The diencephalon contains two structures:

- the thalamus, which acts as a relay station for information passing to the cerebral cortex from the rest of the nervous system
- the hypothalamus, which regulates hormonal, autonomic and other basic body functions such as temperature control, salt and water balance, thirst and appetite.

Within the brainstem, the midbrain controls many sensory and motor functions such as eye movements and coordination of visual and auditory reflexes. Nerve tracts in the pons convey information about movement from the cerebral hemispheres to the cerebellum, which modulates the force and range of muscle movements. Nerve centers in the medulla control digestion, breathing and heart rate.

(a)

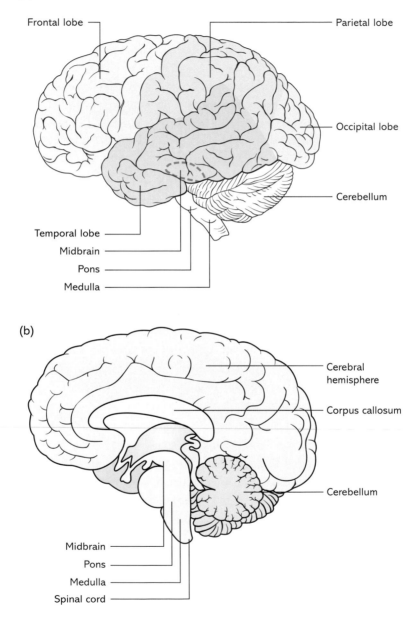

(b)

Figure 1.1 Schematic views of the brain: (a) lateral view; (b) midsagittal section.

Early studies of patients with strokes or other major focal brain injuries revealed that different cortical regions contribute to distinct mental abilities and functions. For example, the frontal lobes are mainly concerned with planning future actions, controlling movements and the abilities associated with self-monitoring and abstract reasoning. The parietal lobes are instrumental in somatic sensation and body image, and in visuospatial reasoning. The occipital lobes are devoted largely to vision. The temporal lobes are often affected by dementing illness and are important for learning and memory, language functions and emotional responses. However, 'parallel processing' is an important organizational principle of brain function. The term implies that when a region or pathway is damaged, others are able to compensate partly for the loss.

Brain cells

In the nineteenth and early twentieth centuries, pioneering neuroanatomists and neuropathologists studied the structures of the brain using careful light microscopic techniques. They identified two characteristic cell types in the brain: neurons (Figure 1.2) and neuroglia.

Neurons, like all cells, are contained within a lipid-bilayer membrane. The fatty acid components of the membrane are oriented with their lipid 'tails' facing inwards towards the opposite layer. Large protein molecules are embedded in or span the membrane and allow structural communication between neurons, and may also be receptors for neurotransmitters or other chemicals that affect cell function. Without such specific 'gateways', drugs must be lipid-soluble to enter brain cells, and hence their rate of entry into the brain depends on their lipid solubility.

Neurons usually have one long process, the axon, which connects with neurons at some distance. They also have many other processes called dendrites that extend like the branches of a tree away from the cell body of the neuron. These dendritic branches form patterns of connections with other neurons that are also typical for that particular area of the brain.

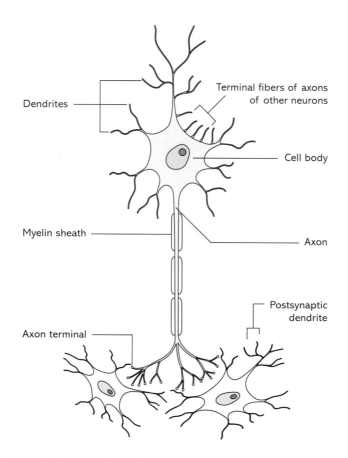

Dendrites

Terminal fibers of axons
of other neurons

Cell body

Myelin sheath

Axon

Postsynaptic
dendrite

Axon terminal

Figure 1.2 Structure of a typical neuron, showing points of contact with cell bodies, axons and dendrites of other neurons.

Internal cell structure. In addition to components common to all cells, within the cytoplasm occur membrane pockets called vesicles or vacuoles, depending on their shape and size. Vesicles often contain chemical neurotransmitters and are typically concentrated close to a synapse ready to release their contents (Figure 1.3). Also, protein threads within the cytoplasm, called microfilaments, function primarily as a supportive system. Microtubules, distinct from microfilaments, are hollow cylindrical protein structures within the cell cytoplasm that:
• provide the cytoskeleton
• help neurons extend long axonal and dendritic processes

- have an important role in transport of materials within the cell, particularly to distant points at the ends of axons and dendrites.

The proteins involved in the assembly of microtubules, called microtubule-associated proteins (MAPs), are abnormal in Alzheimer's disease.

Cell-surface molecules. Large regulatory biomolecules studded in neuron cell membranes are crucial for transfer of information between brain cells and in cell–cell adhesion and recognition. They include:

- *amyloid precursor protein* (APP), a large cell-surface-membrane-spanning protein, important in the biology of Alzheimer's disease

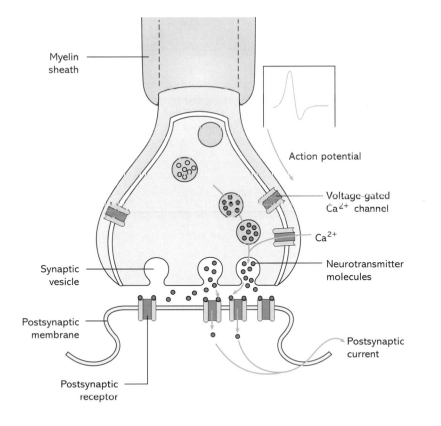

Figure 1.3 Basic mechanism of neurotransmission at a typical synapse.

- *receptors*, i.e. large cell-surface molecules that recognize chemical transmitters released from adjacent neurons. Each receptor recognizes only one type of neurotransmitter, but there may be more than one type of receptor for a single neurotransmitter.

Neuroglia. There are three principal types of glia in the brain.

Astrocytes are star-like cells thought to have a supporting role in the development and maintenance of the nervous system. They appear also to have crucial tasks in the provision of molecular signals to organize brain cell growth, differentiation and repair, and in the organization of brain response to injury.

Microglia are small and round and are the brain's scavenger cells that remove and prepare unwanted material for immune elimination, much as macrophages function outside the blood–brain barrier.

Schwann cells are specialized for production of myelin, the fatty insulation that surrounds the long axons of some larger neurons.

Synapses

Brain cells make complex patterns of connections with each other to form local neural networks, which link together to perform essential brain tasks such as memory or language. These networks adapt to experience by changing their patterns of connections – a phenomenon known as 'synaptic plasticity'.

Communication between adjacent neurons occurs at cell-to-cell junctions called synapses (Figure 1.3). Early neuroscientists recognized the importance of these connections and thought that synapses acted like wiring contacts, passing information in the form of electrical pulses between nerve cells. We now know that electrical synaptic transmission occurs rarely in the nervous system and that most synapses pass information using chemical signals called neurotransmitters.

'Classical' neurotransmitters

Neurotransmitters are contained within vesicles that are typically concentrated close to a synapse ready to release their contents into the synaptic space. Neurotransmitters either excite or inhibit the activity of the target postsynaptic cell. Neurons are classified by the type of neurotransmitter they use to send their signals. The following neurotransmitters are among those implicated in the pathophysiology of brain disorders.

Gamma-amino butyric acid (GABA) functions mainly as an inhibitory neurotransmitter and approximately half of brain cells use it. Disturbance in GABA function can produce devastating effects such as epilepsy.

Glutamate is the principal excitatory neurotransmitter in the brain. Cells that receive glutamate signals can be overstimulated and die (excitotoxicity). Excitotoxic cell death is thought to be an important cause of neurodegeneration in several brain diseases, including Huntington's disease, and may have a role in the dementias of aging such as Alzheimer's disease and vascular dementia.

Acetylcholine has a more specialized function. The cells that synthesize this neurotransmitter have their cell bodies in specific deep brain structures, the nucleus basalis of Meinert (a part of the medial forebrain) and adjacent regions. Their axons project extensively to many higher brain structures, such as the cortex and hippocampi, where the level of transmitter release is probably an important modulating influence on other neural systems, such as those critical for memory and cognition (Figure 1.4). Cholinergic activity is therefore an important modifier of memory function, and it is impaired in Alzheimer's disease.

Peptide neurotransmitters

Until about 25 years ago, it was thought that each neuron used only one transmitter. However, Hokfeldt and colleagues in Sweden have since established the principle of 'coexistence'. They observed that nerve cells could contain both a small-molecule 'classical' neurotransmitter and one of the newly discovered peptide neurotransmitters (consisting of several amino acids ordinarily found in proteins). Peptide transmitters are not only concerned with the control of hormone release by the brain – they also have much more widespread importance. They

13

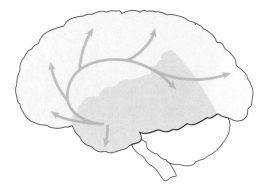

Figure 1.4 Cholinergic projections to the cerebral cortex from the brainstem.

are present at concentrations about one thousandfold less than 'classical' transmitters and are intimately involved in the regulation of the latter's release. Their names usually derive from their endocrine actions: for example, somatostatin (inhibits growth hormone) and corticotropin-releasing factor (stimulates release of adrenocorticotropic hormone, ACTH). Levels of some peptide neurotransmitters are substantially lowered in Alzheimer's disease, and some treatments have been based on attempts to replace them.

Cholinergic neurotransmission

Acetylcholine (ACh) is stored in vesicles at the terminal of a presynaptic cholinergic neuron. When this cell fires, depolarization of the presynaptic terminal membrane opens voltage-dependent calcium channels. Calcium mediates the fusion of vesicles with the presynaptic membrane, resulting in release of ACh into the synaptic cleft by exocytosis (see Figure 1.5). The transmitter molecules then bind to cholinergic receptors on the postsynaptic membrane of an adjacent neuron. This results in any of several processes – for example, activation of ion channels, allowing current flow to spread to adjacent areas of the postsynaptic membrane – which contribute to depolarization of the postsynaptic membrane. Free or bound ACh is quickly broken down by the enzyme acetylcholinesterase into choline and acetate (or the free neurotransmitter may diffuse away into a nearby astrocyte). The choline is reabsorbed into the presynaptic terminal, where it is reprocessed into ACh.

Cholinergic receptors. There are two types of cholinergic receptor:
- muscarinic receptors, which react to muscarine and can be blocked by atropine

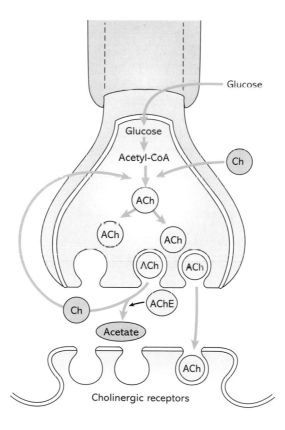

Figure 1.5 Neurotransmission at cholinergic synapses, showing the role of acetylcholinesterase (AChE) in breaking down acetylcholine (ACh) into choline (Ch) and acetate.

- nicotinic receptors, which are activated by nicotine and are not blocked by atropine.

When a nicotinic receptor complex is activated, it changes shape and charge, allowing ions to pass from the outside to the inside of the cell. Activation of a muscarinic receptor results in activation of a 'second messenger' protein within the cell, releasing intracellular calcium and opening nearby potassium channels.

Synaptic plasticity

Even in a healthy brain, patterns of connections between brain cells are not rigid and unchanging but are in a constant state of rearrangement – a phenomenon called 'synaptic plasticity'. Early in brain development there is overproduction of synapses, which are then gradually reduced in number in early adolescence in a process called 'synaptic pruning'. Much later in life there is a more gradual and insidious loss of synapses.

The precise implications of the changes in number of synapses are unknown. However, reduction in synaptic density may reduce the capacity of the brain to respond to experience. There is evidence that synaptic plasticity underpins brain processes as different as memory and brain repair after injury. The brain mechanisms that determine normal development of the nervous system are also thought to be involved in the determination and regulation of synaptic plasticity.

To achieve a perfect relationship between brain information processing and rearrangement of synapses, electrical impulses must be able to influence, in a very precise manner, long-term changes in local neuronal circuit architecture and function. This is probably achieved by regulation of the expression of specific DNA sequences inside the neuronal cell body. In turn, expression of DNA modifies the production of local trophic factors, or the responsiveness of nearby cells to them. These mechanisms probably allow a local group of neurons to 'remember' their exact excitatory or inhibitory patterns of input.

Synaptic plasticity is currently the best hypothesis to explain human memory. Failure to maintain synaptic plasticity as a part of brain aging produces the memory problems typical of healthy old age as well as of the early features of dementia. Generally, synaptic plasticity is a 'necessary' component of memory but it is not established whether alone it provides sufficient explanation of memory. Future interventions for the treatment of dementia will be designed to retain or strengthen the biological mechanisms of synaptic plasticity.

Basic science – Key points

- There are two types of brain cell: the neuron and the glial cell. Neurons do brain work; they process information. Glia support and protect the neurons.
- Neurons communicate at synapses. Most synapses are modified by function, and patterns of synaptic connections are shaped by brain work. This is called synaptic plasticity.
- Most synapses communicate using a chemical transmitter. Acetylcholine is one type of transmitter. It supports brain functions that include learning and memory, through cholinergic transmission.
- The surface of the neuron contains many large molecules involved in cell–cell recognition and adhesion. One of these, amyloid precursor protein, is important in the biology of Alzheimer's disease.
- The internal structure of the neuron is provided by a microtubular cytoskeleton. Special proteins that help assemble the cytoskeleton (microtubule-associated proteins) are abnormal in Alzheimer's disease.

Key references

Engert F, Bonhoeffer T. Dendritic spine changes associated with hippocampal long-term synaptic plasticity. *Nature* 1999;399:66–70.

Eriksson PS, Perfilieva E, Bjork-Eriksson T et al. Neurogenesis in the adult hippocampus. *Nat Med* 1998;4:1313–17.

Kandel ER, Schwartz JH, Jessell TM. *Essentials of Neural Science and Behavior.* Englewood Cliffs, NJ: Prentice Hall, 1995.

Kolb B, Whishaw IQ. *Fundamentals of Human Neuropsychology.* 3rd edition. New York: WH Freeman and Co., 1990.

Maletic-Savatic M, Malinow R, Svoboda K. Rapid dendritic morphogenesis in CA1 hippocampal dendrites induced by synaptic activity. *Science* 1999;283:1923–7.

Anatomy and chemistry of the aging brain

Brain shrinkage. Around age 50, the brain begins to shrink from an average weight of 1.3 kg to about 1.2 kg by the age of 65. Contrary to widespread belief, this shrinkage does not reflect an accelerated loss of nerve cells, but instead results from loss of water and a reduction in the 'normal' complement of brain cells. Some loss of brain substance is nearly universal in aging, but atrophy is much greater in the presence of age-related neurodegenerative disease.

As the brain shrinks with age, the gaps between folds of cortex (sulci) widen and the spaces (ventricles) inside the brain enlarge. In Alzheimer's disease, this cortical shrinkage is more extensive and may be more marked in specific local regions such as temporal or parietal areas. It is not known whether the changes of Alzheimer's disease are categorically distinct from those of 'normal' aging, or whether they represent an exaggeration of these changes.

Magnetic resonance imaging (MRI) reveals the distribution of water within the skull cavity and can thus detect brain shrinkage. When water molecules are subjected to a strong magnetic field, they are induced to resonate and release radio energy. This radiation can be detected by an array of sensors around the head and the sources reconstructed by computer. This reconstruction provides a model of water distribution in the brain. MRI-based maps of normal brain aging are available. These show the need for great care in the interpretation of MRI scans of aging brains (Figure 2.1).

Synaptic and neuronal loss. Coleman and Flood carefully reviewed studies on brain cell loss with aging and challenged the validity of the consensus view that brain cell death is associated with brain aging in the absence of dementia. Later studies showed that, in the absence of dementia, there was no neuronal loss from two brain structures particularly affected by Alzheimer's disease: the hippocampus and the entorhinal cortex. Robert Terry has proposed that the

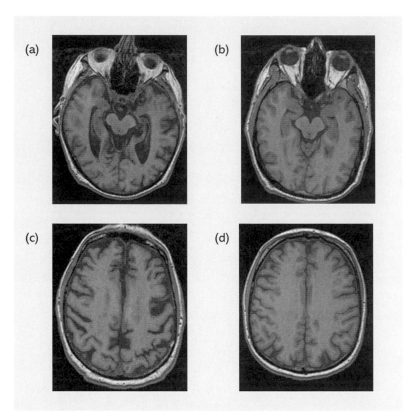

Figure 2.1 Magnetic resonance images of normal and pathologically atrophied brains. Scans (a) and (c) show sulcal widening and/or enlarged ventricles compared with the brains of normal controls shown in scans (b) and (d), respectively. Images courtesy of Dr A Murray, Aberdeen Royal Infirmary, UK.

structural loss of synapses may be the basis of the functional deficits in dementia.

Glucose consumption. The work done by the brain also decreases with age. Although the brain comprises only approximately 2% of the body weight of a 70 kg man, it consumes 20% of his total energy. The metabolic demand of the brain is met by blood flow that is protected at a high and privileged rate compared with other organs. Changes in brain glucose consumption also occur with age. These changes can be measured using positron emission tomography (PET) to chart brain metabolism. PET relies on the simultaneous detection of radiation (positrons) released from short-lived radioactive atoms. As in MRI, detection is achieved by an array of sensors placed around a subject's head. The PET procedure involves rapid synthesis of a very short half-life radiolabeled glucose or other metabolic substrate, injection of the radioactive glucose into an arm vein, and then scanning the head to map the distribution of glucose uptake in the brain.

With aging there are decreases in the amount of glucose taken up by brain cells. Sometimes these decreases can be linked to development of mental symptoms or impairment such as memory decline. Consistent with the pattern of neuropathological lesions in Alzheimer's disease found at postmortem, regional cerebral metabolic studies in vivo show reduced glucose metabolism in the cortical association areas, with relative sparing of the subcortical structures and cerebellum. These reductions are greater the more severe the dementia. Similarly, longitudinal studies show that these changes in regional glucose metabolism precede and may predict later dementia onset.

Neurotransmitters. Levels of specific neurotransmitters decrease gradually with aging. Most neurotransmitter systems show age-related decreases, and there are many indications that these changes correspond to changes in cognitive function. The neurotransmitters involved with control of movement, attention, arousal, the sleep–wake cycle, eating and aggression are all found in discrete brain structures, and neurotransmitter loss caused by disease can often be related to the severity of symptoms associated with these structures.

This principle was first established for dopamine, which is lost in the substantia nigra (a region of the midbrain) of patients with Parkinson's disease. There is a widespread tendency towards loss of dopamine with normal aging, but most individuals suffer only moderate loss and no symptoms appear. In some cases, however, there is dopamine loss of 90% or more and parkinsonian symptoms appear.

Similarly, loss of GABA-releasing cells has been shown in the caudate nucleus of patients with Huntington's disease. The principle is also true for Alzheimer's disease, in which there is a loss of cholinergic neurons projecting from the basal forebrain onto the cortex and hippocampus.

TABLE 2.1

Age- and disease-related abnormalities in neurotransmitter systems

Transmitter/ enzyme	AD	HD	Alc	MID	PD	Aging
Ach-ChAT	↓↓↓	↓	↓	↔	↓	↓
AChE	↓↓	↓	↓	↔		↔
DA	↓	↓	↓		↓	↓
NE	↓		↓	↔		↓↓
GABA	↓	↓	↓			↓
5-HT	↓↓	↑			↓↓	↔
CRH	↓↓				↓	
SS	↓					↔
Glut	↓					↔

AD, Alzheimer's disease; HD, Huntington's disease; Alc, alcoholism; MID, multi-infarct (vascular) dementia; PD, Parkinson's disease; Ach-ChAT, acetylcholine / choline acetyltransferase; AChE, acetylcholinesterase; DA, dopamine; NE, norepinephrine (noradrenaline); GABA, gamma-aminobutyric acid; 5-HT, serotonin; CRH, corticotropin-releasing hormone; SS, somatostatin; Glut, glutamate; ↓, decreased; ↑, increased; ↔, unchanged/uncertain

Other age- and disease-related neurotransmitter abnormalities are shown in Table 2.1.

In general, clinical disease occurs only after extensive loss of neural integrity. This is in accordance with the concept of redundancy or 'brain reserve'. More specifically, the densities of receptors for neurotransmitters are critical determinants of the aging brain's capacity to respond to injury and to pharmaceutical agents.

Microscopic changes with brain aging

Senile plaques are abnormal extracellular structures found in aging brains. They contain the debris of degenerating neurons, called neurites, embedded in an amorphous substance. Early investigators stained affected brain tissue sections and noted that this amorphous substance took up the dyes that stain plant starches, and so the structures were named 'amyloid' plaques (Latin *amylum* for starch). Later biochemical examination showed that this 'amyloid' material was composed mostly of a peptide fragment (variously termed Aβ or β-A4) that is cleaved from a large parent protein molecule (the amyloid precursor protein or APP, see Chapter 7). In the aging brain, senile plaques can be found at various stages of 'maturation' ranging from diffuse deposits of amyloid to the complex neuritic lesions described above (Figure 2.2). Currently, two main types of senile plaque are recognized.

- Diffuse plaques are made up of filamentous material and poorly structured material. These do not correlate with dementia severity.
- In contrast, neuritic plaques contain dense bundles of amyloid fibrils and are subdivided into classical (with a dense core) and primitive neuritic plaques (without this core).

Amyloid is a novel substance, which the body's immune system may well recognize as foreign. Not surprisingly, in reaction to amyloid the microglia (the small glial cells that function as the brain's 'scavengers') may be stimulated to intense metabolic activity. Cellular respiration consumes oxygen and generates highly reactive oxygen-containing 'free radicals'. Harmful products

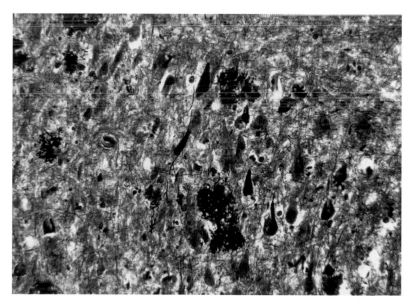

Figure 2.2 Brain tissue containing senile plaques and neurofibrillary tangles. Von Braunmuhl stain. Image reproduced by courtesy of Dr J Mackenzie, Aberdeen Royal Infirmary, UK.

of cell oxidative damage caused by free-radical attack can activate microglia by binding to their cell-surface receptors. Detailed biochemical analysis of markers of microglial activation provide evidence that a low-grade inflammatory response occurs in the aging brain, which could explain why sustained use of non-steroidal anti-inflammatory drugs (NSAIDs) may reduce the risk of Alzheimer's disease (see Chapter 7).

Neurofibrillary tangles (NFTs, Figure 2.2) are made up of abnormal aggregates of neurofilaments, and under the electron microscope appear as pairs of 10 nm diameter filaments arranged to form a double helix. The lesions probably originate as inclusions within the living neuronal cell body and are essentially biochemical modifications of the natural neuronal cytoskeleton. When neurons die in Alzheimer's disease and related conditions, NFTs are found between surviving neurons and have been likened to 'ghosts' or 'gravestones' of their deceased hosts.

Contemporary neurobiologists have investigated NFT formation in health and disease using powerful molecular biological and genetic techniques. A key constituent of the tangle is derived from a naturally occurring microtubule-associated protein called tau. Normally, several of the tau amino acids contain phosphate groups. In Alzheimer's disease, tau is hyperphosphorylated, making it more likely to aggregate into paired helical filaments and tangles. Alternatively, tau proteins can combine with glucose (glycation) as a result of oxidative stress linked to age-related abnormal glucose metabolism. Glycated tau can promote the formation of paired helical filaments. When deposition of NFTs becomes more extensive and involves the brain structures essential for memory, symptoms of Alzheimer's disease are probably inevitable.

Functional changes with brain aging

The common structural changes described previously are probably responsible for several changes in mental abilities as people age.

Slowed mental processing is the most frequently detected age-related change in brain function. Reaction time, which is a simple test of the time taken to respond to a defined stimulus, slows from early adulthood onwards. Most of this slowing occurs in the central and not the peripheral nervous system, and is more apparent in complex mental tasks.

Several mechanisms may account for mental slowing:

- Synaptic loss may slow information processing by depriving the brain of its multiplicity of neuronal interconnections.
- Degradation of the myelin sheath may slow information flow by decreasing the speed of signals in long bundles of axons. Such degradation is probably caused by age-related free-radical oxidation of fatty acids in the myelin in a process called membrane lipid peroxidation. Myelin peroxidation is present in all brain cells examined from middle age onwards.
- Oxidative changes may also affect the large regulatory biomolecules in neuronal membranes.

Each of these age-related changes is a plausible cause of mental slowing, but a causal relationship has not been proven for any of them. Since mental slowing and myelin peroxidation are universal with aging, they are most probably linked.

Selective cell loss in key brain structures

The hippocampus is critical to memory function. Brain cell numbers in the hippocampus are typically preserved in old people, even in the presence of memory problems before death. It was previously thought that brain cell loss in the hippocampus was the principal cause of memory impairment in 'normal' old age. However, we now know that the hippocampus does not lose brain cells as an inevitable consequence of aging. Instead, substantial hippocampal cell loss is a sign of neurodegenerative disease.

The frontal lobes are strongly affected by aging, and there is now a consensus that several psychological changes (mostly decline) with aging reflect deterioration of these structures. Unfortunately, it is impossible to know the precise role of the frontal lobes in aging because of their size and complexity. Like the rest of the cortex, the frontal lobes do not function symmetrically. Instead, one side is 'dominant' over the other. Also distinct anatomic regions in the frontal lobes appear to be affected unequally by aging processes.

The dorsolateral frontal cortex evolved last in brain development and is particularly vulnerable to age-related changes. This observation has encouraged some to believe that the most recently evolved areas of the cortex are affected most by aging and Alzheimer's disease.

In normal old age, there is also selective loss of forebrain cholinergic cells in humans, monkeys and rats. The extent of acetylcholine loss has been shown to be closely related to the decline of memory function in normal old people. However, decreasing acetylcholine transmission does not fully explain the loss of cognitive functions in old age. Many other transmitters and peptides are also involved. In general, the cortex is not particularly vulnerable to aging but its communicating subcortical structures seem to be so. Also, some specific transmitter systems may be more affected than others.

'Successful' aging

An increase in the proportion of old people without significant chronic disabilities is one of the success stories of modern geriatric medicine. Where mild-to-moderate degrees of cognitive decline were previously attributed simply to 'old age', now this is no longer assumed. Instead, the contribution of poor general physical health to cognitive decline in old age is now widely recognized. With adequate care, such a decline in health is often avoidable. Disease-free elderly often show considerably less decline in cognitive abilities than was commonly considered the norm for their age. These individuals demonstrate the importance of maintaining general health for 'successful' aging. A number of common medical conditions can impair cognition in the elderly and thus are appropriate intervention targets with a view to maintaining full cognitive capacity into old age (Table 2.2).

Brain aging and dementia: what makes the difference?

The conventional view among physicians is that there are well-established neuropathological changes that ensure an easy distinction between dementia – particularly Alzheimer's disease – and normal aging without dementia. Currently, all neuropathological systems agree on the appearance of the brain in 'classical' Alzheimer's disease, but there is

TABLE 2.2

Medical conditions that can impair cognition in old age

Common	Rare
• Infection	• Inflammatory
− bronchopneumonia	− sarcoidosis
− urinary tract infection	− systemic lupus erythematosus
• Cardiorespiratory	
− myocardial infarction	• Metabolic disorders
− congestive heart failure	• Trauma
− atrial fibrillation	− subdural hematoma
• Nutritional	
− vitamin deficiency	
• Endocrine	
− hypothyroidism	
− hypocalcemia	
− diabetes mellitus	
• Neoplasia	
− most tumors	

much uncertainty about the precise boundaries between dementia and aging. Classical Alzheimer's disease is characterized by extensive neuronal death sufficient to explain a reduction in brain weight by about 35%, widespread accumulation of senile plaques and formation of NFTs. Granulovacuolar degeneration and Hirano bodies are also detectable.

Essentially, because senile plaques and NFTs occur in aging without dementia, most pathologists rely on the extent and location of these features to confirm a clinical diagnosis of dementia. The reasons for linking pathology to clinical state seem obvious but do little to support the acceptance of neuropathological criteria as a gold standard for Alzheimer's disease, having little value in diagnostically difficult or 'early' cases. Standardized neuropathological criteria for Alzheimer's disease are of two types.

- One, like those of the Consortium to Establish a Registry for Alzheimer's Disease (CERAD), is based on a combination of clinical information and an age-related senile plaque score. The validity of these criteria remains poorly documented.
- Another approach is best exemplified by Braak and Braak, who have suggested criteria derived from their observations on the progression of NFT formation in the cerebral cortex. The Braak and Braak scheme proposes that, in the early development of dementia, NFTs are detected in the transentorhinal cortex, with only slight changes in the hippocampus (Stages I and II). The neocortex does not become involved until Stages III and IV, when changes already present become more severe. In Stages V and VI, NFT formation extends into the neocortex and is more severe in the hippocampus.

Currently, studies are underway to develop consensus criteria that combine the CERAD and Braak and Braak approaches to dementia definition and will be of value in clinically difficult cases. Longitudinal observational studies of cognitive aging, with postmortem examination, may solve this problem. So far, they reveal a highly complex problem where the boundaries between aging and dementia reflect individual

The aging brain – Key points

- In the absence of dementia, brain shrinkage is normal after age 50. It is largely explained by loss of water, not by brain cell death.
- Clinical severity of dementia symptoms is related to loss of transmitters, especially acetylcholine.
- Senile ('amyloid') plaques are present with aging in the absence of dementia. Neurofibrillary tangles and loss of synaptic density are more strongly associated with dementia.
- With aging there is mental slowing, attributable to reduced synaptic efficiency and degradation of information transfer systems inside the brain.
- Age-related changes in the frontal cortex probably explain most cognitive impairment with aging in the absence of dementia.

variation in the brain's response to neuronal aging. Additional contributions from aging of the cerebral vasculature and the effects of late-acting genetic repair mechanisms are also involved. Controversially, the resources available to withstand brain aging (the 'cerebral reserve') may account for some of the differences between individuals in their capacity to withstand similar degrees of brain pathology.

Key references

Barger SW, Harmon AD. Microglial activation by Alzheimer amyloid precursor protein and modulation by apolipoprotein E. *Nature* 1997;388:878–81.

Braak H, Braak E. Evolution of neuronal changes in the course of Alzheimer's disease. J *Neural Transmission* 1998;53(suppl): 127–40.

Davis DG, Schmitt FA, Wekstein DR, Markesbery WR. Alzheimer neuropathologic alterations in aged cognitively normal subjects. *J Neuropathol Exp Neurol* 1999; 58:376–88.

Flood DG, Coleman PD. Neuron numbers and sizes in aging brain – comparisons of human, monkey and rodent data. *Neurobiol Aging* 1988;9:453–63.

Green MS, Kaye JA, Ball MJ. The Oregon brain ageing study: neuropathology accompanying healthy ageing in the oldest old. *Neurology* 2000;54:105–13.

Harman D. A theory based on free radical and radiation chemistry. *J Gerontol* 1956;11:298–300.

Jellinger KA, Bancher C. Neuropathology of Alzheimer's disease: a critical update. *J Neural Transm Suppl* 1998;54:S77–95.

Kirkwood BL, Wolff SP. The biological basis of ageing. *Age Aging* 1995;24:167–71.

Mouton PR, Martin LJ, Calhoun ME et al. Cognitive decline strongly correlates with cortical atrophy in Alzheimer's dementia. *Neurobiol Aging* 1998;19:371–7.

Perry G, Raina AK, Nunomura A et al. How important is oxidative damage? Lessons from Alzheimer's disease. *Free Radic Biol Med* 2000; 28:831–4.

Ritchie K, Kildea D. Is senile dementia 'age-related' or 'ageing-related'? – evidence from meta-analysis of dementia prevalence in the oldest old. *Lancet* 1995;346:931–4.

Samuel W, Masliah E, Hill LR et al. Hippocampal connectivity and Alzheimer's dementia – effects of synapse loss and tangle frequency in a two-component model. *Neurology* 1994;44:2081–8.

Von Dras DD, Blumenthal HT. Dementia of the aged: Disease or atypical-accelerated aging? Biopathological and psychological perspectives. *J Am Geriatr Soc* 1992;40:285–94.

Wolf DS, Gearing M, Snowdon DA et al. Progression of regional neuropathology in Alzheimer disease and normal elderly: findings from the Nun study. *Alzheimer Dis Assoc Disord* 1999;13:226–31.

In neurodegenerative illness, brain changes at the molecular, subcellular, cellular or tissue levels can reach a threshold level of severity, such that cognitive capacities are lost. Some such conditions, for example Alzheimer's and Parkinson's disease, may arguably represent exaggerations of the 'normal' aging process, but many certainly do not.

The 'threshold–decompensation' model of symptom formation applies to many organ systems and can be applied to cognitive decline (Figure 3.1). In normal development, cognitive capacities grow through infancy and childhood so that optimal functional capacity is attained in early adulthood (left-hand, ascending portion of curve). The measure of this optimum cognitive capacity may be influenced not only by genes but also by childhood illnesses, education, nutrition, or exposure to neurotoxins. Exposure to severe harmful influences may limit brain

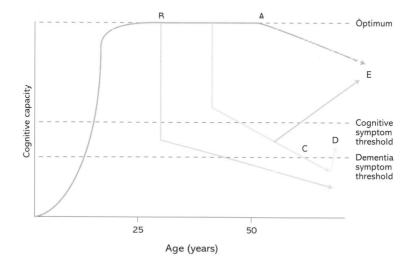

Figure 3.1 Trajectories of cognitive development and decline (see text for explanation).

development so that optimum functional maturity is not attained, as is seen in neurodevelopmental disorders. Upon attaining optimum development, the 'normal' cognitive capacity curve typically begins to decline slowly, several decades after reaching its optimum, at about age 50 (A). A catastrophic event (B) such as a traumatic brain injury or stroke can suddenly reduce cognitive capacities beyond the critical symptom threshold, below which cognitive symptoms appear. Such injury can result in lasting cognitive disability, but some injuries may be insufficient to cause an observable cognitive syndrome. These less severe injuries may still reduce the brain's cognitive reserve such that the 'normal' aging trajectory now proceeds from a lower starting point (green line). Accelerated decline in the trajectory now crosses the dementia symptom threshold in relatively early old age (C). With treatment or recovery, functional integrity may be re-established, leading to a partial recovery (D) or complete restitution of capacities (E). If some residual damage remains, however, the trajectory will begin at a lower point on the cognitive capacity axis and so the dementia symptom threshold will be approached or crossed sooner.

Cognitive disorders: delirium, dementia and focal syndromes

Insults to the functional capacity of the brain can result in different cognitive syndromes. Fulminant neurodegenerative processes (rarely) or severe alterations of the brain's metabolic milieu (more commonly) can provoke *delirium*. Slow neurodegenerative processes or more chronic injury states typically provoke *dementia*. Though these syndromes share the cardinal feature of global cognitive decline, they are otherwise distinct.

Delirium. The hallmark of delirium is clouding of consciousness. Other common features include abnormalities of emotion, perception and behavior, as well as cognition. The terms 'delirium' and 'confusion' are sometimes used interchangeably when clouding of consciousness produces changes in mental capacities. The term 'delirium' has a more precise meaning than 'confusion', and the former is preferred.

Two important aspects of consciousness are:

- level of arousal (from coma to stupor to normal vigilance and beyond)
- ability to alter or focus one's attention at will and to discriminate among several simultaneous environmental stimuli.

In delirium, a reduced ability to perceive and distinguish among competing stimuli may result in reduced capacity to focus attention on a task at hand, to sustain that attention, or to move it at will to another task. Abnormal visual phenomena are also common and may include misinterpretation of visual stimuli (illusions) or visual perception in the absence of an appropriate stimulus (hallucinations). Delirium usually develops over a period of hours, tends to fluctuate in severity, and may be interspersed with periods of normality. A delirious patient's world is often colored by emotional responses to distorted experiences. Intense fear or panic may result from bizarre or threatening visual hallucinations. Such visual symptoms, the characteristic fluctuating course, and the patient's preoccupation with their own inner world are useful clues to the presence of delirium.

Delirium is typically provoked by an abnormality in the metabolic substrate required for normal brain function. The clinician's task is therefore to identify the provoking cause such as poisoning or electrolyte imbalance. When identified, such causes are often reversible, and successful treatment usually results in symptomatic improvement. However, delirium can be among the most vexing of all conditions to treat. Often, despite diligent efforts, the provoking toxic or metabolic derangement cannot be identified and therefore treated. In this case, conservative and supportive care must be offered in the hope that the condition will resolve spontaneously.

Delirium has a complex relationship with the types of chronic progressive brain disease that typically provoke dementia. Chronic progressive brain disease does not necessarily provoke alterations in consciousness. Thus, the course of these diseases may not include delirious states. Occasionally, healthy people may develop delirium when they become severely physically ill, but pre-existing brain disease increases vulnerability to delirium. This pre-existing disease may or may not be severe enough to have provoked dementia. When delirium is superimposed on dementia, the clinical picture may be perplexing.

New occurrence of delirium may be an early indicator of such a brain disease, but it may also signal the presence of a severe but previously unsuspected medical illness. The case fatality rate with delirium is substantial, though much improved with modern care, and therefore onset of delirium is a warning sign that requires immediate attention. Other outcomes include full recovery or sustained insult to the brain and dementia. Upon recovery from delirium, patients with pre-existing dementia will revert to a clinical appearance of uncomplicated dementia.

Dementia. Sometimes, particularly in the UK, the term 'dementia' is used to signify a brain disease with a precise corresponding neuropathology. However, we prefer to define dementia as a clinical syndrome characterized by a decline in multiple aspects of cognition, and not attributable to any alteration in consciousness. Symptoms may include impairment in:

- memory
- reasoning
- language
- perceptual interpretation
- ability to deal with visuospatial relationships
- personal judgment
- 'praxis', the usually extra-conscious ability to order and coordinate movements or activities to achieve some simple goals such as walking or writing
- gnostic function, the ability (usually taken for granted) to interpret cognitively what is adequately perceived in any of the five primary sensory modalities.

Two neuropsychiatric classification systems, DSM-IV and ICD-10, define dementia broadly in this way, but apply somewhat different operational terms. Both systems require a decline in memory and other abilities of a degree sufficient to interfere with everyday activities. The ICD-10 also requires alteration in personality, while DSM-IV specifically mentions apraxia, aphasia (loss of language abilities), agnosia (difficulties in interpretation of a perception, e.g. failure to recognize a familiar face), and problems in executive functioning (planning, organizing, sequencing, abstracting). The DSM-IV criteria for dementia of the Alzheimer's type are given in Table 3.1.

Dementia is sometimes taken to imply irreversibility, and it is true that most dementing illnesses are incurable. However, irreversibility is not a defining feature. A number of specific causes of dementia provoke a fully or at least partially recoverable state (Table 3.2). Indeed, a thorough search for the causes of dementia, including specifically reversible causes, is essential. It is no longer acceptable medical practice – if it ever was – to consign a patient with 'dementia' to the dustbin of medical nihilism.

Focal cerebral disorders. The most common focal presentations are associated with large strokes. There is, however, another group of cognitive disorders that result from more circumscribed focal brain injury. These disorders are characterized by loss in one, or at most two, cognitive domains such as language (aphasia) or interpretation of perception (agnosia). Therefore, they cannot be defined as dementia, which requires a more global decline in cognition. Because the provoking lesions are relatively static, changes in mental ability attributable to the lesioned area can be distinguished from the general consequences of traumatic brain injury (which tend to improve or heal over time). Typical psychological symptoms linked to particular regions of the brain may be conveniently divided among the frontal lobes, parietal lobes, temporal lobes and occipital lobes (Table 3.3).

Frontal lobes. Lesions of the frontal lobes produce some of the most significant symptoms of focal cerebral disease. Removal of frontal lobe function produces either an apathetic state or an opposite disinhibition with overexpansive behaviors, social intrusiveness and loss of social and moral control. Errors of judgment in all fields of human endeavor occur in such patients. Sometimes there is a change in temperament, seen by someone who knows the patient well as an empty or fatuous cheerfulness without meaning or significance. The ability to maintain attention or carry out sequential planned activities may also be affected.

TABLE 3.1

DSM-IV diagnostic criteria for dementia of the Alzheimer's type

A. The development of multiple cognitive deficits manifested by both

(1) memory impairment (impaired ability to learn new information or to recall previously learned information);

(2) one (or more) of the following cognitive disturbances:

(a) aphasia (language disturbance)

(b) apraxia (impaired ability to carry out motor activities despite intact motor function)

(c) agnosia (failure to recognize or identify objects despite intact sensory function)

(d) disturbance in executive function (i.e. planning, organizing, sequencing, abstracting).

B. The cognitive deficits in criteria A1 and A2 each cause significant impairment in social or occupational functioning and represent a significant decline from a previous level of functioning.

C. The course is characterized by gradual onset and continuing cognitive decline.

D. The cognitive deficits in criteria A1 and A2 are not due to any of the following:

(1) other central nervous system conditions that cause progressive deficits in memory and cognition (e.g. cerebrovascular disease, Parkinson's disease, Huntington's disease, subdural hematoma, normal-pressure hydrocephalus, brain tumor)

(2) systemic conditions that are known to cause dementia (e.g. hypothyroidism, vitamin B_{12} or folic acid deficiency, niacin deficiency, hypercalcemia, neurosyphilis, HIV infection

(3) substance-induced conditions.

E. The deficits do not occur exclusively during the course of a delirium.

F. The disturbance is not better accounted for by another Axis 1 disorder (e.g. major depressive disorder, schizophrenia).

TABLE 3.2

Specific causes of dementia that provoke a fully or partially recoverable state

Cause	Treatment
Depressive illness	Antidepressants, electroconvulsant therapy, psychotherapy
Drug intoxication	Supportive therapy, specific antidotes occasionally
Normal-pressure hydrocephalus	Surgical shunt
Infective illness	Antibiotics
Neoplasia	Steroids for any associated edema
Cardiovascular disease	Specific therapy to correct hypertension, ischemia, etc.
Subdural hematoma	Surgical evacuation
Metabolic/endocrine	Specific corrective therapy

Parietal lobes. Lesions of either parietal lobe typically cause visuospatial and topographical difficulties or agnosia. Visuospatial problems may be detected during clinical examination by asking the patient to produce or copy simple drawings, such as a cube or clock face, or to construct simple patterns from matchsticks. Topographical problems become apparent when the patient has difficulty in negotiating a new environment, for example being unable to find the way out, or getting lost or stranded in familiar surroundings. When the dominant parietal lobe is affected, complex language defects may appear, including alexia (inability to read) and agraphia (inability to write). Motor coordination may also be disturbed. Non-dominant parietal lobe lesions disturb awareness of body image and its relation to external space. Parietal lobe disease in dementing illnesses can cause dressing apraxia (inability to conceptualize or execute the routine task of putting on clothes in the correct orientation or in appropriate order) or various forms of agnosia.

Temporal lobes. Lesions of the dominant temporal lobe typically cause language problems, which may include both expressive and sensory aphasia (the inability to create language or interpret it). Lesions of the non-dominant temporal lobes tend to show fewer signs or symptoms. Within the inferomesial portions of the temporal lobes lie the hippocampus and parahippocampal structures, which are critical for memory; when these areas are lesioned bilaterally, memory loss can be devastating. Interestingly, unilateral lesions in these regions are completely 'silent' or produce isolated loss of certain memory aspects.

TABLE 3.3

Functions subject to localized cortical impairment

Frontal lobe

- Responsiveness and involvement (apathy)
- Response inhibition ('disinhibition')
- Movement planning
- Task sequencing, planning and organization

Parietal lobe

- Somatosensory integration
- Tactile form recognition
- Visual perception
- Spatial relations
- Language (mostly receptive and interpretive)
- Praxis
- Motor coordination

Temporal lobe

- Auditory processing
- Visual processing
- Verbal memory
- Language (mostly expressive)

Occipital lobe

- Visual recognition

Symptoms and signs – Key points

- The cerebral reserve hypothesis proposes that brain disease or damage must exceed a reserve of cerebral ('cognitive') capacities before cognitive symptoms are detectable.
- Delirium is characterized by clouding of consciousness, and disturbances of emotion, perception and behavior. It tends to fluctuate in severity and may be interspersed with episodes of normality. It is often reversible, but complex associations with chronic progressive brain disease are common.
- Dementia is a clinical syndrome that is not attributable to a disturbance of consciousness, where impaired memory is always present and other symptoms or signs (e.g. visuospatial deficits) may be present.
- Reversible ('treatable') causes of delirium and dementia must be identified in the early investigation of cognitive impairment in old people.
- Localized cortical impairment is often associated with specific cognitive deficits related to the specific functions of the area of impaired cortex (e.g. parietal lobe damage is linked to visuospatial deficits).

Lesions in more anterior temporal lobe structures, such as the amygdala, can also cause persistent disturbances in temperament and the control of aggressive impulses. Unlike other focal brain lesions, injuries to the temporal lobe, particularly if they extend deep into its structure, can produce a characteristic visual-field defect. This is caused by damage to the temporal radiation of fibers that convey visual information from the brainstem to the occipital lobes. If the visual-field defect is present with dementia, it indicates a focal brain lesion, for example a tumor, and suggests that the dementing illness may be caused by the lesion.

Occipital lobes. All of the symptoms of occipital lobe lesions are linked to the important role of this brain region in visual functions. Symptoms range from 'cortical blindness' to a less dramatic inability to read while the ability to write is retained (alexia without agraphia), or failure to identify colors or objects. The occipital lobes are not usually involved in neurodegenerative dementing illnesses.

Personality changes

As with cognitive capacity, personality may change with increasing age, either as a result of 'normal' developmental processes or as a reflection of brain disease. In healthy aging, personality traits are typically quite stable with the exception that many elderly people become more preoccupied with their own mental life. If there is a stereotypical personality change with aging, it is decreased impulsivity, fear of sudden change, and preoccupation with orderliness. These features of 'normal' aging may be exaggerated by higher life expectancy among inflexible, stronger personality types, causing over-representation of this type among the very old. There are also contemporary trends towards a greater sense of individuality with age, and blurring of gender roles (men become more nurturing and women more achievement oriented). If personality changes deviate from the above, or are out of keeping with earlier traits, it is likely that such changes reflect an underlying brain disease. Indeed, personality change can sometimes herald the later emergence of a frank dementia syndrome.

Key references

Bergener M. *Psycho-Geriatrics. An International Handbook.* New York: Springer,1988.

Evans JG, Williams TF. *Oxford Textbook of Geriatric Medicine.* Oxford: Oxford University Press, 1992.

Kaplan HI, Sadock BJ. *Concise Textbook of Clinical Psychiatry.* Derived from Kaplan and Sadock's Synopsis of Psychiatry. 7th edition. Baltimore: Williams and Wilkins, 1996.

Light LL, Burke DM. *Language, Memory, and Aging.* Cambridge: Cambridge University Press, 1988.

Lishman WA. *Organic Psychiatry. The Psychological Consequences of Cerebral Disorder.* Oxford: Blackwell Scientific, 1987.

Although the neurodegenerative diseases that cause dementia characteristically attack cortical and subcortical structures essential for cognition, their effects are not limited to these regions. Other areas of the brain, responsible for mood or emotional responsivity or for regulation of neurotransmitters such as dopamine or norepinephrine, are commonly affected. If these regions are diseased, patients with dementia commonly develop non-cognitive psychiatric symptoms such as hallucinations and delusions, disturbance of mood, or various troublesome behavioral anomalies. Generally, these symptoms may be categorized using terms familiar to psychiatrists for the description of psychopathology in other mental illnesses. Such symptoms usually cause considerable distress to patients and especially to their carers, to the point that they can be decisive determinants of need for placement or other urgent intervention.

Delusions and hallucinations

A delusion is an unshakable belief that is implausible, idiosyncratic and fully embraced by the patient. Delusional beliefs are common in dementing illness. Though dementia patients may have difficulty describing their delusions or affirming their fixed quality, the characteristically persistent and pervasive nature of delusions is often revealed by the patient's recurrent behavior. Typical delusions in dementia include the idea that one's home is not one's own, or that a spouse or carer has been replaced by a stranger. Sometimes, the delusion appears to serve the purpose of making good or explaining a deficit in memory; for example, mislaid or forgotten household items may become the subject of delusional beliefs that a thief has entered the home and taken the items. Even if someone else later locates the 'stolen' item, the demented patient remains unconvinced and may remark on how cunning the 'thief' was to replace the item before his capture.

Hallucinations are sensory perceptions that occur without adequate stimulus. These can occur in any of the five primary sensory modalities.

Visual hallucinations, common in delirium but rare in other psychiatric conditions, occur fairly often in dementia. Frequently, these are part of complex hallucinatory phenomena involving several senses simultaneously, for example both vision and hearing. The content of hallucination in dementia is often threatening or perplexing to the patient, provoking agitated or troublesome behavior. Persistent or recurrent hallucinations of a single form may also engender secondary delusional beliefs; for example repeated visions of a deceased spouse may lead the sufferer to believe that the spouse is still alive. More fragmentary hallucinations, often prompted by normal visual perceptions, are also common in dementia. These visual phenomena include the perception of animals, 'microbes' on food, and visits by

Case report 1

Mrs H, aged 82, was visited by a nurse at home. Her daughter who lived a few houses away was also present. Mrs H complained that men had entered her home and taken things during the previous few months. Items 'stolen' included mementoes from her husband, a photograph album and a broken antique clock. In fact, she said, she had caught the men only the other night and that the police had come and arrested them. Her daughter explained that her mother had simply 'mislaid' some of the items (they were all easily found by her grandson) and that the clock had been sent for repair. The alleged episode with the men and police reflected events of a few nights previously when Mrs H had walked to her daughter's house in an agitated state, stating that men were fighting in her living room and that the police were there. The grandson noted that this account fitted events in a police program on the television. 'Mom', said the daughter, 'it was the television you were watching. A police story. Now, don't worry. Just sit down, and have you remembered to lock up and bring your keys?' The mother replied that she had, and handed her daughter the remote control for the television.

> **Case report 2**
>
> Mrs B was a 74-year-old who had been widowed 2 years previously. Recently her neighbors had become concerned by her leaving the apartment block at about 2 a.m. to go 'shopping for my husband's dinner'. At home assessment she had many features of dementia. Her routine included repeatedly cleaning and pressing her husband's old clothes, preparing meals for him and identifying to observers where she saw him in the room. Unusually, she had placed a framed photograph of him at his place at the dining table. The cover glass had been removed from the photograph and the area around his mouth was worn thin by her kissing and trying to press food through an aperture she had made.

strangers with whom a conversation is remembered but never witnessed. Visual hallucinations are particularly characteristic of Lewy body dementia and frequently have an illusory quality, being triggered by otherwise neutral stimuli such as a wallpaper pattern or crumpled bed sheet. Hallucinations are rarely described by demented patients without some delusional elaboration.

Mood abnormalities

Dementing illnesses sometimes first appear with clinical symptoms of depression, and depressed mood is a common feature of Alzheimer's and several other common neurodegenerative diseases, including Parkinson's disease, and stroke. Patients with insight may feel sad or despondent about their loss of cognitive abilities, but this reaction is less common than might be surmised. More common are depressive changes with 'endogenomorphic' features, such as psychomotor slowing or apathy, disturbed sleep and appetite, self-neglect or self-reproach, and nihilistic ideas of impoverishment or physical illness. The common concurrence of dementia syndromes and clinical depression can occasionally create diagnostic challenges, but depressive features should be treated regardless of whether they are secondary to a neurodegenerative disorder. Other dementia patients may show agitation, excessive worry or arousal, or exaggerated fears. All of these mood states may motivate a variety of untoward or troublesome behaviors that can hugely increase the burden or complexity of care.

Behavioral disturbances

Behavioral disturbances in dementia may be conveniently subdivided into new and unwanted behaviors, or the disappearance or neglect of normal and desired behaviors. New behaviors can often be attributed to the presence of hallucinations or delusions. Similarly, aggression and irritability can sometimes be linked to abnormal persecutory ideas. In contrast, some repetitive or stereotyped behaviors can be traced to over-learned or over-rehearsed occupational or domestic tasks. A severely demented mailman, for example, may wander a regular route around his residential home mailing pieces of newspaper into unlikely crevices. Typically, it is the new behaviors, which derive from psychosis or altered perception of reality, that are most likely to improve with carefully monitored, low-dose neuroleptic therapy.

Although new behaviors such as aggression and wandering are troublesome, the disappearance of old behaviors can sometimes be even more distressing to family or friends. Behavioral deficits can extend across a wide range of activities including dressing, use of sanitary facilities, or eating. As dementia progresses, carers can be surprisingly resourceful in developing compensatory strategies. Self-care routines, though tiresome for a daughter with a demented mother, can sometimes become playful or even humorous. Placing an electric kettle on a gas hob is never funny, however, and loss of domestic skills poses a frequent hazard to the health and safety of the patient and others.

Neuropsychiatric complications – Key points

- Neuropsychiatric complications can be extremely important determinants of the ability of individuals with dementia to live with only minimal to moderate assistance.
- Delusions and hallucinations are frequent in dementia. When compelling, they can be among the most troublesome neuropsychiatric complications, necessitating closer management.
- Low mood may occur at any stage of dementia, but often responds to antidepressant treatment. The diagnosis of depressive disorder in a person with dementia is complicated by coexistent symptoms of the dementia such as disturbance of language or perception.
- Behavioral disturbances in dementia may be grouped as new, unwanted behaviors (e.g. aggression) or failure to perform desired behaviors (e.g. loss of domestic skills).

Key references

Cumming JL. The Neuropsychiatric Inventory: assessing psychopathology in demented patients. *Neurology* 1997;48(suppl 6):S10–16.

Frisoni GB, Rozzini L, Gozzetti A et al. Behavioral syndromes in Alzheimer's disease: description and correlates. *Dement Geriatr Cogn Disord* 1999;10:130–8.

Katona C, Levy R. *Delusions and Hallucinations in Old Age.* London: Gaskell / Royal College of Psychiatrists, 1992.

Kaufer DI, Cummings JL, Christine D et al. Assessing the impact of neuropsychiatric symptoms in Alzheimer's disease: the Neuropsychiatric Inventory Caregiver Distress Scale. *J Am Geriatr Soc* 1998;46:210–15.

Lovestone S, Howard R. *Depression in Elderly People.* London: Martin Dunitz, 1996.

Clinical history

The most important part of any clinical evaluation is the history, usually obtained from the carer or other well-informed third party.

The examiner must first seek and document evidence that the patient's present state represents a decline from a prior level of abilities. The natural history of the illness (prodrome, onset, course, prominent symptoms) is recorded. Was disease onset insidious, as is usual in Alzheimer's disease, or sudden as in a stroke? Did symptoms progress smoothly and inexorably, typical of Alzheimer's disease, or in a pattern of stepwise decline suggesting a vascular process? Specific symptoms are sought for their differential diagnostic significance. If the patient has been ill for several years, has he developed the prominent difficulties with language, praxis or gnostic functions that are typical of Alzheimer's disease?

The medical history can be equally informative and must not be overlooked. Are there risk factors for cerebrovascular illness, such as diabetes, atrial fibrillation, poorly controlled hypertension or generalized atherosclerosis? Are features of Parkinson's disease present, such as slowed movements and mentation, tremor, difficulties with phonation or gait disturbance? Have these responded to treatment, for example with L-dopa? Also, is there any significant history of alcohol misuse or exposure to other toxins?

Physical and routine laboratory examination

Approximately 5% of old people with apparent early dementia have an underlying physical illness which, when treated, effectively improves their mental function (see Table 3.2). Most of these conditions are revealed, at least in part, by careful physical examination, and the sensitivity and specificity of the physical findings can be enhanced by routine laboratory tests. A complete physical and neurological examination is therefore essential, and the following tests should be performed routinely:

- blood pressure measurement
- auscultation for carotid bruits
- chest auscultation
- hematology, including differential cell count and ESR (optional)
- biochemistry (calcium and phosphate, thyroid function tests and simple urinalysis)
- renal (creatinine, BUN) and hepatic function (ALT, serum albumin) tests.

Low-cost metabolic screening (glucose and electrolytes) is also useful, but routine cerebrospinal fluid examination is not recommended.

Mental status examination

This may be divided into examination of the cognitive deficit proper and other associated emotional or behavioral features. It is essential to test basic cognitive capacities. Otherwise, a patient with early dementia may fool the examiner by maintaining a competent 'social demeanor' and concealing their deficits with approximate answers, bantering or changes of topic.

Mini Mental State Examination (MMSE). For all but the most severely ill, cognitive mental state can be readily assessed using a brief, standardized inventory of cognitive capacities such as the MMSE. The MMSE is brief and simple enough for use in routine office practice with older patients, yet is sufficiently comprehensive that when combined with other clinical measures it provides a valuable index of dementia severity and staging (Table 5.1).

The MMSE probes five different cognitive 'domains'. The first section covers orientation, memory and attention. Memory is tested by noting the number of trials required to learn three object names then testing recall later. Attention is tested by the serial subtraction of 'sevens' from one hundred or spelling the word 'world' backwards. The next questions test for loss of ability to:
- repeat a simple spoken phrase (language fluency)
- name common objects (nominal aphasia)
- follow a three-stage verbal command (receptive aphasia, apraxia)
- comprehend and follow a one-stage written command (alexia)

- write a sentence spontaneously (agraphia).

The test is completed by asking the patient to copy a simple figure of two intersecting pentagons (constructional apraxia). The maximum score is 30 points, and a score of less than 24 is broadly indicative of cognitive impairment. However, this threshold is not universal – individuals of lower original mental ability are likely to achieve lower scores, whereas those with superior intellect will typically do better. For example, for a university graduate a score of 27 or less would probably suggest cognitive impairment.

National Adult Reading Test (NART). This is another simple test, designed for completion by a carer, doctor or nurse, to estimate original mental ability. The patient is asked to read a standard list of words with irregular spellings. For example, someone who had not encountered the word 'syncope' might be unaware of the conventional emphasis placed on the last letter. The test comprises 50 such words of decreasing familiarity. It can be administered quickly and correlates well with original intelligence quotient.

Short Blessed test of activities of daily living, or the Dementia Symptom Rating Scale (DSRS). These assess a patient's ability to carry out routine daily activities that require an intact cognitive apparatus.

Briefer mental tests for non-specialist use. The MMSE can be shortened for use in primary care with little loss of specificity. Items retained in the short version include:

- orientation to day of the week
- spell the word 'world' backwards
- recall three words after a delay of 1 minute with distraction
- the request to write a proper sentence.

Another reliable indicator of dementia is a carer's account of deterioration in four activities of daily living, including:

- managing medication
- using the telephone
- coping with a budget
- using transport.

TABLE 5.1

Mini Mental State Examination (MMSE) questions

1. **Orientation**

    (Score 1 for correct, 0 for incorrect)
    What is the year we are in?
    What season is it?
    What is today's date?
    What day of the week is it today?
    What month are we in?
    What county are we in?
    What country are we in?
    What town are we in?
    Can you tell me the name of this place?
    What floor of the building are we on?

2. **Registration**

    Ask the subject if you may test his memory. Then say the names of
    3 unrelated objects, clearly and slowly, about one second for each,
    'lemon, key, ball'. after you have said all 3, ask him to repeat them. The
    first repetition determines his score (0–3) but keep saying them until he
    can repeat all 3, up to 5 trials. If he does not eventually learn all 3,
    recall cannot be meaningfully tested. (Score 0–3)

3. **Attention and calculation**

    Ask the subject to begin with 100 and subtract 7 from 100 and keep
    subtracting 7. Stop after 5 subtractions (93,86,79,72,65). Score the
    total number of correct answers. Ask the subject to spell the word
    'world' backwards. The score is the number of letters in correct order
    (e.g. dlrow = 5, dlorw = 3). The highest score will be recorded.
    (Score 0–5)

4. **Recall**

    Ask the subject if he can recall the 3 words you previously asked him
    to remember. (Score 0–3)

5. **Naming**

    (a) Show the subject a wristwatch and ask him what it is.

    (b) Repeat for a pencil.

    (Score 0–2)

TABLE 5.1 (CONTINUED)

6. **Repetition**

Ask the subject to repeat this sentence after you: 'No Ifs, Ands, or Buts'. Allow only one trial. (Score 0–1)

7. **Three-stage command**

Have the subject follow this command: 'Take a paper in your hand, fold it in half, and put it on the floor'. Score one point for each part correctly executed. (Score 0–3)

8. **Reacting**

On a blank piece of paper print the sentence 'Close your eyes' in letters large enough for the subject to see clearly. Ask him to read it and do what it says. Score one point only if he actually closes his eyes. (Score 0–1)

9. **Writing**

Give the subject a blank piece of paper and ask him to write a sentence for you. Do not dictate a sentence, it is to be written spontaneously. It must contain a subject and a verb and be sensible. Correct grammar and punctuation are not necessary. (Score 0–1)

10. **Copying**

On a clean piece of paper, draw intersecting pentagons, and ask him to copy it exactly as it is. All 10 angles must be present, and 2 must intersect to score one point. Tremor and rotation are ignored. (Score 0–1)

Maximum score: 30

Source: *J Psychiatr Res* 1975;12:189–98

These eight items can be easily incorporated into a routine domiciliary consultation, together with the clock-drawing test, which also has good sensitivity and specificity for dementia (Figure 5.1). It is strongly recommended that family physicians use and record these formal cognitive test procedures as a minimum in their evaluation of dementia,

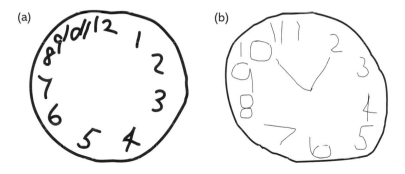

Figure 5.1 The clock-drawing test. (a) Exaggerated spacing of low numbers leads to crowding of high numbers. (b) The patient was instructed to 'Draw a clock face and set the hands to ten past eleven'. Number 12 is missing.

particularly when evaluating and monitoring pharmacological dementia treatments (see Chapter 8).

Assessment of delirium or altered consciousness. Informal quantitative assessment of attention and concentration may be particularly useful for detection of delirium. Another valuable test is to ask the patient, if cooperative, to extend both arms, then fully dorsiflex the hands and hold this awkward posture. The clinician may demonstrate, or even assist the patient to achieve the desired posture, but then lets go. Delirious patients, not only those with hepatic encephalopathy, often exhibit asterixis, or irregular myoclonic jerking movements either of the entire hand or of selected digits.

Assessment of disordered emotion and behavior. There is good evidence that behavioral and emotional concomitants of dementia are as important as cognitive state in predicting burden of care, need for residential placement, etc. Several instruments have therefore been introduced recently to enable comprehensive and uniform assessment of behavioral symptoms in dementia.

The Neuropsychiatric Inventory (NPI) introduced by Cummings and colleagues is the best known of these. It is a structured interview for administration to a carer or other party who is familiar with the patient's behavioral repertoire. It has ten sections covering hallucinations, delusions, agitation/anxiety, depressed mood, apathy, irritability or aggressive behaviors, stereotyped or repetitive purposeless behaviors, resistiveness to care, and socially inappropriate behaviors. Each section includes a 'probe' question to be asked verbatim. Positive responses are followed up with specific questions intended to elaborate specific behaviors, and then further questions are asked to establish the frequency and severity of these behavioral difficulties. A final panel of questions inquires about changes in sleep, appetite, energy level, and expressed sexual interests.

Diagnostic imaging

Consensus groups have not previously recommended routine structural imaging using CT or MRI in the early investigation of dementia, but these procedures have been recently recommended, if available. In specialty settings these investigations reveal cortical atrophy, white matter changes, space-occupying lesions and vascular disease, including areas of ischemia and/or infarction. Unless extensive, atrophy is of uncertain value in the diagnosis of dementia (see Figure 2.1). In the absence of dementia, white-matter lesions may be associated with cognitive deficits including slowed processing, immediate and delayed memory and overall impairment of planning and mental function.

PET or, more commonly, single photon emission computed tomography (SPECT) are of diagnostic value, particularly for clinically distinguishing between Alzheimer's disease and cerebrovascular dementia. With specialized modification, such as high-resolution imaging of medial temporal thickness or volumetric measures, MRI or PET and SPECT techniques are potential markers of dementia progression and the effects of antidementia drugs.

Clinical examination and investigations – Key points

- Initial assessment must include a careful clinical history and investigations to detect causes of reversible ('treatable') dementia.
- All initial assessments should record an estimate of dementia severity and be based on a method for which age- and education-standardized normal ('non-demented') values are available.
- In community-based clinical practice, simple formal tests of cognitive function and activities of daily living should be performed and recorded. In specialist practice, standardized behavioral and emotional ratings should be used routinely.
- SPECT and other metabolic imaging may help distinguish between Alzheimer's disease and predominantly vascular dementia. The place of brain structural imaging techniques in the routine assessment of dementia is uncertain.

Key references

Berg L, McKeel DW Jr, Miller JP et al. Clinicopathologic studies in cognitively healthy aging and Alzheimer's disease: relation of histologic markers to dementia severity, age, sex and apolipoprotein E genotype. *Arch Neurol* 1998;55: 326–35.

Grut M, Jorm AF, Fratiglioni L et al. Memory complaints of elderly people in a population survey: variation according to dementia stage and depression. *J Am Geriatr Soc* 1993;41:1295–300.

Heinik J, Reider-Groswasser II, Solomesh I et al. Clock drawing test: correlation with linear measurements of CT studies in demented patients. *Int J Geriatr Psychiatry* 2000;15:1130–7.

Jagust W, Thisted R, Devous MD Sr et al. SPECT perfusion imaging in the diagnosis of Alzheimer's disease: a clinico-pathologic study. *Neurology* 2001;56:950–6.

Knopman DS, DeKosky ST, Cummings JL et al. Practice parameter: Diagnosis of dementia (an evidence-based review). Report of the Quality Standards Subcommittee of the American Academy of Neurology. *Neurology* 2001;56:1143–53.

Konno S, Meyer JS, Terayama Y et al. Classification, diagnosis and treatment of vascular dementia. *Drugs Aging* 1997;11:361–73.

Lund and Manchester Groups. Clinical and neuropathological criteria for frontotemporal dementia. *J Neurol Neurosurg Psychiatry* 1994;57: 416–18.

Mathuranath PS, Nestor PJ, Berrios GE et al. A brief cognitive test battery to differentiate Alzheimer's disease and frontotemporal dementia. *Neurology* 2000;55:1613–20.

McKeith IG, Gakasji D, Kosaka K et al. Consensus guidelines for the clinical and pathologic diagnosis of dementia with Lewy bodies (DLB): report of the consortium on DLB international workshop. *Neurology* 1996;47:1113–24.

McKhann G, Drachman D, Folstein M et al. Clinical diagnosis of Alzheimer's disease: report of the NINCDS-ADRDA Work Group under the auspices of Department of Health and Human Services Task Force on Alzheimer's Disease. *Neurology* 1984;34:939–44.

Nathan J, Wilkinson D, Stammers S, Low JL. The role of tests of frontal executive function in the detection of mild dementia. *Int J Geriatr Psychiatry* 2001;16:18–26.

Pasquier F. Early diagnosis of dementia: neuropsychology. *J Neurol* 1999;246:6–15.

Patten J. *Neurological Differential Diagnosis.* 2nd edition. New York: Springer, 1996.

O'Brien J, Barber R. Neuroimaging in dementia and depression. *Advances in Psychiatric Treatment* 2000;6:109–19.

Roman GC, Tatemichi TK, Erkiunjuntti T et al. Vascular dementia: diagnostic criteria for research studies. Report of the NINDS-AIREN International Workshop. *Neurology* 1993;43: 250–60.

Royal College of Psychiatrists. Consensus statement on the assessment and investigation of an elderly person with suspected cognitive impairment by a specialist old age psychiatry service. *Council Report* CR49, 1995 [currently being updated].

Waldemar G, Dubois B, Emre M et al. Diagnosis and management of Alzheimer's disease and other disorders associated with dementia. The role of neurologists in Europe. European Federation of Neurological Societies. *Eur J Neurol* 2000;7:133–44.

Walstra GJM, Teunisse S, vanGool WA et al. Reversible dementia in elderly patients referred to a memory clinic. *J Neurol* 1997;244:17–22.

Increased survival after onset of symptoms is one of the reasons why the prevalence of dementia is increasing throughout the world. With improved nursing care and more widespread use of antibiotics to treat intercurrent infections, individuals now commonly survive 10 years or longer with dementia. This was not always the case – in the 1950s, the pioneering geriatric psychiatrist Sir Martin Roth and colleagues used distinctions in duration of illness to show that dementia differed from other severe psychiatric syndromes, notably depression, in the elderly. At that time, most old people hospitalized with dementia in the UK survived approximately 2 years; those with depression survived longer. The increasing prevalence of dementia that has resulted from longer survival after disease onset has been cited by the late American epidemiologist Ernest Gruenberg as one of several 'failures of success' – a phrase he coined to describe advances in practice that, paradoxically, result in an increased burden of disease. Incidentally, the same unfortunate principle applies to treatments that slow progression (and therefore delay death) in established cases of Alzheimer's disease or other dementias.

Alzheimer's disease is by far the most common cause of the dementia syndrome in the Western world. With the exception of cerebrovascular disease, which is apparently more common in Japan than elsewhere, other causes are relatively rare and account for only a few percent of cases. Table 6.1 shows the relative frequencies of the various illnesses that underlie prevalent dementia in Europe and North America. It can be seen that dementia often has multiple causes, and the combination of Alzheimer's disease with cerebrovascular disease in particular is more frequent than would be predicted if the two were unrelated. The common concurrence of Alzheimer and vascular pathology has lead to debate concerning the relative frequencies of these two diseases because investigators tend to give different emphasis to one or the other at diagnosis.

TABLE 6.1

Causes of dementia

- Alzheimer's disease (50%)
- Mixed Alzheimer–vascular diseases (20%)
- Cerebrovascular disease (10%)
- Dementia with Lewy bodies (10%)
- 'Reversible' causes* (5%)
- Unknown cause (5%)

*See Table 3.2

Risk factors for dementia and Alzheimer's disease

Age is the key risk factor for dementia. The condition is rare in young or middle-aged adults but, driven mainly by the age-specific incidence of Alzheimer's disease, which doubles approximately every 5 years until age 85, dementia becomes extremely common in old age. Between the ages of 75 and 80 years (a typical age at death for those who have survived to a nominal retirement age of 65), more than 5% of people develop dementia. Yet, contrary to popular belief reflected in the term 'senility' or 'senile dementia', age itself is not a cause of dementia. Many very old people have intact cognition – an observation that supports the principle that association does not imply cause. In Figure 6.1a, (i) and (ii) depict identical neurodegenerative processes in two individuals with substantially different cognitive capacities in early life. Individual (i) starts with less cerebral reserve, so his trajectory crosses the symptom threshold a few years earlier, i.e. this person experiences earlier onset (and higher age-specific risk) of Alzheimer's disease. Figure 6.1b shows the effect of various forms of apolipoprotein E, a cholesterol transport protein with normal variants that predict different onsets and age-specific risks for Alzheimer's disease (see Chapter 7). These variants also predict the trajectory in middle age of cognitive abilities or of early metabolic and anatomical brain features predicted by this model of Alzheimer's disease. Figure 6.1c suggests the possible effects of environmental risk or protective factors that can

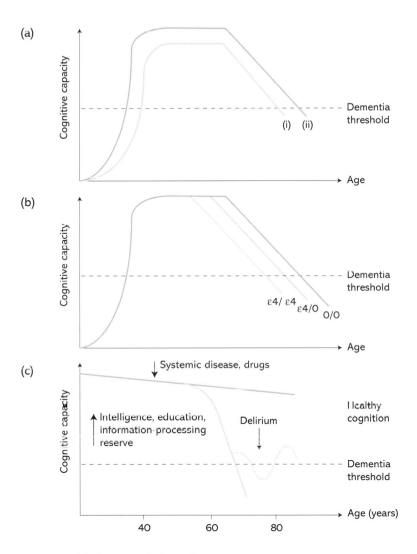

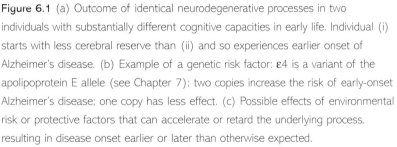

Figure 6.1 (a) Outcome of identical neurodegenerative processes in two individuals with substantially different cognitive capacities in early life. Individual (i) starts with less cerebral reserve than (ii) and so experiences earlier onset of Alzheimer's disease. (b) Example of a genetic risk factor: ε4 is a variant of the apolipoprotein E allele (see Chapter 7); two copies increase the risk of early-onset Alzheimer's disease; one copy has less effect. (c) Possible effects of environmental risk or protective factors that can accelerate or retard the underlying process, resulting in disease onset earlier or later than otherwise expected.

accelerate or retard the underlying process, resulting in disease onset earlier or later than otherwise expected (exaggerated or attenuated age-specific risk).

Sex. All prevalence studies show women are more often affected by dementia than are men. Typically, in most health services, there are twice as many demented women as men known to the service. This is only partly explained by better life expectancy among women because, even when this is taken into account, a slight excess of women remains. Recent studies from Europe and the USA have shown that this small increase reflects a strong disproportion in the incidence of Alzheimer's disease among women after age 85. With increasing life expectancy, one should therefore expect a still greater excess of women with Alzheimer's disease. Some of this excess may be caused by impaired neuronal function and neuronal protective mechanisms with estrogen depletion after menopause. Social factors (e.g. widowhood) may also exacerbate the apparent disability associated with dementia in older women. There is some evidence that profound decreases in gonadal steroid production disrupt neuronal function and impair neuronal protective mechanisms. More likely, social and biologic aging processes act together to increase the burden of disability in old women for whom the added burden of age-related cognitive impairment leads to decompensation of adaptive processes.

Family history. Individuals whose first-degree relatives (parents, siblings or children) have Alzheimer's disease show an approximate threefold increased risk of developing Alzheimer's disease compared with those who lack such a family history. This increase holds across the spectrum of ages. Thus, person A who has an affected sibling may have three times the risk of person B who does not, whether both A and B are aged 65 or 85; however, the absolute risks at the later age are much higher: an 85-year-old person without a family history will be at higher risk than a 65-year-old with an affected relative.

Although Alzheimer's disease tends to run in families, the majority of present-day cases of Alzheimer's disease do not have an affected relative. This is because familial predisposition to Alzheimer's disease is expressed mainly in very late old age. Fewer than half of predisposed individuals develop the disease before age 85. Therefore, the absence of a family history may reflect nothing more than the absence of sufficient numbers of very old relatives to reveal the familial tendency toward the disease.

However, it is worth noting that a tendency towards clustering in families is insufficient to allow us to conclude that a disease is inherited. If that were so, we could conclude that tendencies to become a physician were inherited traits because a large proportion of the sons and daughters of doctors pursue careers in medicine! In general, a genetic trait, such as a tendency towards disease, will produce familial aggregation, but we cannot infer the former from the latter. Hypotheses about the genetic causes of Alzheimer's disease are discussed in the next chapter.

Race and geography. Among African-Americans, the higher prevalence of vascular dementia is usually attributed to the higher prevalence of cardiovascular risk factors and lower socioeconomic status of this vulnerable group. Specifically, around 25% of Americans are hypertensive, but the age-adjusted prevalence of hypertension among African-Americans is about 33%. Large differences in the proportion of dementia attributable to vascular dementia are reported between Asia and Europe. There are about 17 patients with Alzheimer's disease to every 10 with vascular dementia in Europe, whereas in Japan there are about 17 cases of Alzheimer's disease for every 34 of vascular dementia. Comparisons between ethnically homogenous Japanese populations in Japan, Hawaii and Washington State in the USA are also informative. As populations have migrated, so has the ratio of Alzheimer cases to vascular cases of dementia reversed.

The Indianopolis–Ibadan dementia project has identified important differences between the African-Americans of Indianapolis and the Yoruba of Ibadan in Nigeria. Early studies were confounded by large differences in the age structure of the two communities, but recent analyses of incident cases show that age-standardized incidence rates for both dementia and Alzheimer's disease are about two- to threefold lower in Ibadan than in Indianapolis. These findings, and others from cross-cultural studies in those of Japanese and African ancestry, strongly suggest that environmental factors, probably acting with specific genes, make important contributions to the causes of Alzheimer's disease. Possible environmental factors include diet, alcohol intake, smoking and exercise.

Vascular pathology. Vascular lesions can exaggerate the clinical effects of Alzheimer pathology, so that strokes and other vascular changes act as a 'risk factor' for the onset of dementia in those developing Alzheimer's disease. Important risk factors for such vascular pathology, and indeed for vascular dementia, are:
- poorly controlled hypertension
- diabetes mellitus
- hyperhomocysteinemia
- hyperlipidemias
- smoking
- various indices of an individual's general tendency towards atherosclerosis.

Much less is known about the epidemiology of other rarer causes of dementia than about the epidemiology of Alzheimer's disease and vascular dementia. With the possible exception of Lewy body dementia (an entity that borders controversially with Alzheimer's disease in some cases and with Parkinson's disease in others), none of these rarer conditions accounts for more than a few percent of dementia cases. As is true of Alzheimer's disease, their incidence (particularly the incidence of vascular dementia) increases among the very old. Their relationship to age is much weaker, however, than that of Alzheimer's disease. As a result, the older the population, the greater the relative frequency of Alzheimer's disease as a cause of dementia. Figure 6.2 shows the increase with age in the proportion of dementia caused by Alzheimer's disease. You can see that, at age 65, Alzheimer's disease typically represents about half of all dementias, but by 85 years the proportion has increased to well over three-quarters. Many people now live to age 85, so the greatest public health concern is Alzheimer's disease.

Hyperhomocysteinemia. Homocysteine is an amino acid that is a key intermediate in the metabolism of sulfur-containing amino acids.

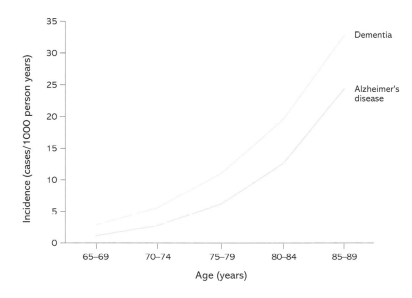

Figure 6.2 The age-specific incidence of moderate-to-severe dementia and Alzheimer's disease in Europe and the USA (adapted from Jorm AF, Jolley D 1998). The figure suggests a growth with age that is more or less exponential between the ages of 65 and 85, with the rate doubling every 5 years. Thereafter, the increase may slow somewhat. If milder cases are included, the rates are approximately double those depicted.

Conversion of homocysteine to methionine or cysteine is by folate / vitamin B_{12}, so their deficiency produces hyperhomocysteinemia. This is easily corrected by folate / vitamin B_{12} supplementation. The relative risk of vascular disease in subjects from the top quintile of total plasma homocysteine is about twice that of subjects in the lower four quintiles. This risk is multiplicative with other risk factors like smoking and hypertension. Possible mechanisms to explain increased risk include impaired renal function caused by atherosclerotic disease. In these terms, hyperhomocysteinemia could be as much a consequence of vascular disease as its cause; however, follow-up studies in the UK and USA support the hypothesis that elevated plasma homocysteine is an antecedent of vascular disease and not its consequence.

Several studies have shown an inverse relationship between plasma homocysteine and cognitive function in late life. Current estimates suggest that 8–10% of age-related cognitive variation can be safely attributed to homocysteine. Case-control studies show greater plasma homocysteine in Alzheimer's disease than in non-demented old people but, as in vascular disease, this could be as much a consequence of poor nutrition in dementia as a causal factor. The Framingham follow-up study has provided compelling evidence that increased homocysteine is a relevant risk factor for Alzheimer's disease. After adjustment for the presence of other known risk factors (age, sex, vascular risk factors, plasma folate/B_{12} and apolipoprotein E genotype), plasma homocysteine predicted the later onset of dementia in non-demented old people followed up for 1–11 years. Figure 6.3 shows the cumulative incidence of dementia in those subjects in the highest quartile of plasma homocysteine (> 13.2 µmol/L). Possible mechanisms to explain increased dementia risk linked to homocysteine include its known

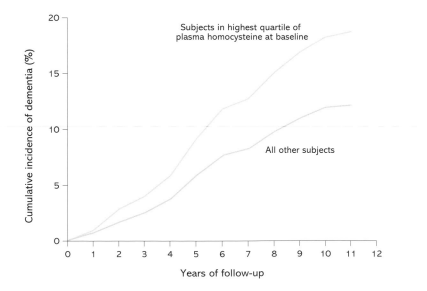

Figure 6.3 Cumulative incidence of dementia in those subjects in the highest quartile of plasma homocysteine (> 13.2 µmol/L). Adapted from Seshadri et al. 2002.

oxidative potential to damage neuronal membranes and DNA and its capacity to sensitize neurons to the harmful effects of amyloid.

Folic acid and vitamin B_{12} supplementation will lower homocysteine by about 25–35% in hyperhomocysteinemia. The extent of reduction is partly modified by a polymorphism in the methylenetetrahydrofolate reductase (MTHFR) gene and by the dose of folate. Clinical trials to prevent or postpone dementia onset in at-risk individuals by homocysteine lowering are currently underway.

Other risk and possible protective factors for Alzheimer's disease. It is clear that not all people experience a similarly increased risk as they age. For example, those who have suffered moderate-to-severe head injury, sufficient to cause an hour's loss of consciousness or amnesia, are probably at increased risk. By contrast, people of higher intelligence or greater educational attainment are at reduced risk. The reasons for this are not completely understood, but a reasonable explanation portrays Alzheimer's disease as a chronic neurodegenerative process that begins many years before the onset of dementia itself (Figures 3.1 and 6.1). It includes a long latent stage that may last for several decades, as well as a prodromal phase that probably accounts for much but certainly not all of the phenomenon of mild age-related cognitive decline. Those with more 'cerebral reserve' suffer more neurodegeneration before symptoms of dementia become evident. This previously noted concept of 'cerebral reserve' may explain why low educational level appears as a risk factor for Alzheimer's disease. In most cultures, educational attainment is highly correlated with intelligence and with synaptic density. The few studies that have attempted to separate the highly correlated attributes of intelligence and education suggest that the former 'drives' the relationship between education and the risk of Alzheimer's disease, though this remains controversial.

Other environmental influences may also slow the progression of the Alzheimer process. Notably, these influences are thought to act principally in the latent or prodromal states of this process, so that their effect is a delay in the age at which dementia symptoms appear. The benefit of the several factors that may achieve such delay seems to be

63

limited to a critical time window, that is, the effect may disappear a variable number of years before dementia symptoms would otherwise occur. Among several possible protective influences, the following are now thought to be most promising.

- Hormone replacement therapy among postmenopausal women. The benefit of this intervention may disappear as long as 10 years prior to onset of dementia symptoms.
- Sustained use of non-steroidal anti-inflammatory drugs. Here the benefit seems to disappear about 2 years prior to dementia onset, that is, about the time patients begin to show the first prodromal symptoms of Alzheimer's disease. The available evidence suggests that full anti-inflammatory doses offer no improvement in their protective effect over low, analgesic doses.
- Antioxidant vitamin supplements. Antioxidants are the only interventions shown in large trials to produce a disease-modifying effect *after* dementia symptoms are evident, and their benefits for prevention may be sustained longer than the other interventions described here.
- Possibly, histamine-H2-blocking agents or 'statin' drugs.

Note that none of these interventions has yet been demonstrated to be effective in definitive randomized trials, so that their benefit is not proven. Instead, these factors may give rise to interventions that may reduce the risk of Alzheimer's disease in the future (see Chapter 9). One intriguing report has also suggested that regular consumption of red wine is associated with reduced risk of Alzheimer's disease. Red wine contains antioxidant flavonoids that, together with antioxidant vitamins, may have a direct neuroprotective activity. Red wine is also thought to protect against cardiovascular, and therefore perhaps cerebrovascular, disease and may reduce the risk of Alzheimer's disease by attenuating the influence of these known risk factors.

Epidemiology of the dementing illnesses – Key points

- Alzheimer's disease is the commonest form of dementia in the Western world. Elsewhere, vascular and reversible ('treatable') types of dementia may be somewhat more frequent.
- Race and geography contribute to differences in incidence of dementia, suggesting that environmental factors – possibly nutritional – may be important.
- Age is the most important risk factor for Alzheimer's disease. Family history, cerebrovascular disease and hyperhomocysteinemia are relevant but less important than age.
- Some medicines and nutrients may slow the progression of Alzheimer's disease. These include non-steroidal anti-inflammatory drugs, hormone replacement therapy (when used in the decades following menopause), antioxidant vitamin supplements, and possibly statins, antihypertensive medicines and histamine-H2-blocking drugs.

Key references

Christensen H, Korten AE, Jorm AF et al. Education and decline in cognitive performance: compensatory but not protective. *Int J Geriatr Psychiatry* 1997;12:323–30.

Fratiglioni L, Ahlbohm A, Viitanen M, Winblad B. Risk factors for late-onset Alzheimer's disease: a population-based, case-control study. *Ann Neurol* 1993;33:258–66.

Galanis DJ, Petrovitch H, Launer LJ et al. Smoking history and middle age and subsequent cognitive performance in elderly Japanese-American men. The Honolulu-Asia Aging Study. *Am J Epidemiol* 1997;145:507–15.

Gao S, Hendrie HC, Hall KS, Hui S. The relationships between age, sex, and the incidence of dementia and Alzheimer disease: a meta-analysis. *Arch Gen Psychiatry* 1998;55: 809–15.

Jick H, Zornberg GL, Jick SS et al. Statins and the risk of dementia. *Lancet* 2000;356:1627–31.

Jorm AF, Jolley D. The incidence of dementia: a meta-analysis. *Neurology* 1998;51:728–33.

Ott A, Stolk RP, van Harskamp F et al. Diabetes mellitus and the risk of dementia. The Rotterdam Study. *Neurology* 1999;53:1937–42.

Perrig WJ, Perrig P, Stähelin HB. The relation between antioxidants and memory performance in the old and very old. *J Am Geriatr Soc* 1997;45: 718–24.

Plassman BL, Welsh KA, Helms M et al. Intelligence and education as predictors of cognitive state in late life: A 50-year follow-up. *Neurology* 1995;45:1446–50.

Prince MJ, Bird AS, Blizzard RA, Mann AH. Is the cognitive function of older patients affected by antihypertensive treatment? Results from 54 months of the Medical Research Council's trial of hypertension in older adults. *BMJ* 1996;312:801–5.

Seshadri S, Beiser A, Selhub et al. Plasma homocysteine as a risk factor for dementia and Alzheimer's disease. *N Engl J Med* 2002;346(7):476–83.

Zandi PP, Carlson MC, Plassman BL et al. Hormone replacement therapy and incidence of Alzheimer disease in older women. The Cache County Study. *JAMA* 2002;288:1–7.

Zandi PP, Breitner JCS. Do NSAIDs prevent Alzheimer's disease? And if so why? The epidemiological evidence. *Neurobiol Aging* 2001;22:811–17.

Genetics

For decades it was thought that rare, early-onset variants of Alzheimer's disease were 'familial' and probably genetic, while the common, later-onset types were 'sporadic'. The familial forms most often showed the characteristics that about half of the offspring of a given case would themselves develop Alzheimer's disease. Males and females appeared equally vulnerable. An example pedigree of this type is shown in Figure 7.1. The usual explanation for such familial aggregation is that the predisposition to disease is transmitted by a single copy of a

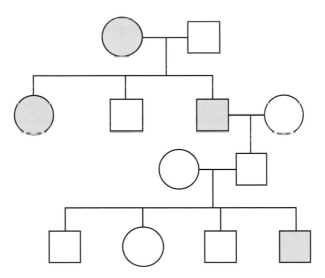

Figure 7.1 A pedigree showing the distribution of Alzheimer's disease cases (filled symbols) among male (squares) and female (circles) members of successive generations. Both sexes are affected at similar rates, and there is no preferential transmission from fathers or mothers. About one half of the offspring of each case (and thus about one half the brothers or sisters of any affected individual) will themselves develop the disease.

defective gene located on one of the 22 chromosomes (autosomes) other than the x and y sex chromosomes.

Not all cases of early-onset (< 65 years) Alzheimer's disease show the sort of familial aggregation seen in Figure 7.1, but about half do. In the past 10 years mutations at three genes have been found to provoke this sort of early-onset familial Alzheimer's disease. These genes probably account for between a third and half of pedigrees like those in Figure 7.1. The remainder are presumably caused by other genes. The first discovered 'Alzheimer's gene' is in the Down's syndrome region of chromosome 21 and encodes a lengthy protein molecule that can be cleaved near its N-terminus to yield the Aβ peptide. The precise functions of this amyloid precursor protein (APP) are still under investigation, but it is known to span the neuronal membrane, having a long cytoplasmic domain, a short and lipophilic transmembrane domain, and a relatively short extracellular domain. Figure 7.2 shows

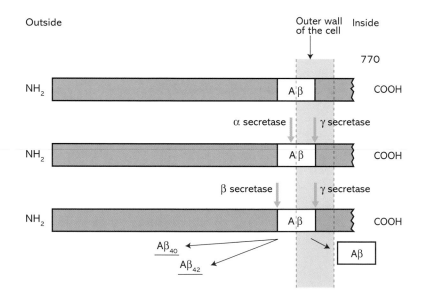

Figure 7.2 The amyloid precursor protein (APP) embedded in a neuronal membrane. The critical Aβ fragment is at the junction of the transmembrane domain of the molecule and its extracellular domain. Three different enzymes are thought to cleave APP in different ways.

how APP spans the membrane. The Aβ fragment resides at the junction of the transmembrane domain and the extracellular domain. Several different point mutations in or adjoining the coding region for the Aβ fragment are now known to provoke the Alzheimer's disease phenotype. A number of other nearby mutations appear to be harmless. The critical role of the pathogenetic mutations is to promote cleavage patterns that produce intact Aβ peptide. The inevitable appearance of Alzheimer's disease in individuals with pathogenetic APP mutations is some of the strongest evidence for the role of Aβ in the causation of Alzheimer's disease.

The two other known 'Alzheimer's genes' are mutations of novel proteins that are called 'presenilins' because they again are subject to rare mutations that can provoke early-onset ('presenile') familial Alzheimer's disease. The two genes, *PS-1* and *PS-2* on chromosomes 14 and 1, respectively, are strongly homologous and are probably descendants of a single progenitor gene. Most *PS-1* mutations cause Alzheimer's disease with an even earlier onset characteristic (usually in the 40s) than is seen with the pathogenetic *APP* mutations. *PS-2* mutations have a more variable effect, provoking onsets in the 50s–70s. Notably, both the presenilin-1 and presenilin-2 proteins are believed to play an important role in the processing of APP and in amyloidogenesis. Their discovery has only served to strengthen support for the importance of the role of Aβ in Alzheimer's disease pathogenesis – even though the exact role of Aβ remains controversial. There is some evidence to support the possibility that γ secretase (Figure 7.2) is a presenilin.

The importance of these three genes lies in the clues they provide to the causal mechanisms of Alzheimer's disease. It should be stated clearly, however, that they are not important causes of Alzheimer's disease (a very common illness) because they are exceedingly rare. Probably no more than 10% of presenile Alzheimer's disease results from these mutations, and the figure is much smaller (< 1%) for Alzheimer's disease overall. The mutations are therefore of enormous biological interest but almost no public-health interest, because most Alzheimer's disease occurs in later life and has a much less distinctive pattern of familial aggregation.

As discussed previously, the evidence for genetic causes of Alzheimer's disease extends well beyond the phenomena of the rare, early-onset familial variants. Familial aggregation in Alzheimer's disease is strong, even when onset is (typically) late. There are problems here in discerning the true extent of familial aggregation: when the 'fore-ordained' onset is in late old age, many predisposed relatives will die of other, unrelated causes before expressing their predisposition by developing Alzheimer's disease. This problem may be dealt with by using a technique called 'survival analysis'. This is a statistical approach that attempts to adjust for the effects of mortality from other causes by considering only those relatives who have survived to a particular age. Survival analyses have shown, for instance, that a first-degree relative (brother, sister or offspring) of someone with well-diagnosed Alzheimer's disease will him/herself have a 40–50% chance of developing Alzheimer's disease if they live beyond age 90. Similar methods suggest that the comparable risk among first-degree relatives of unaffected population 'control' subjects is about 15%. Both figures are probably underestimates, reflecting difficulty in ascertainment of dementia in elderly relatives, many of whom are long deceased. The risk to relatives of Alzheimer's disease cases is therefore increased about threefold (the same as the risk based on epidemiological inquiry).

How much of this risk is genetic, and how much is acquired through shared environment? Answers to this sort of question are available through the study of twin pairs. Although all twins are born at the same time and are typically reared in circumstances where they share many of their early environmental influences, monozygotic (MZ) and dizygotic (DZ) twin pairs differ importantly in their biology. Twin studies compare the degree of similarity within MZ and DZ pairs, typically also comparing this with similarity among random pairings of unrelated individuals. If there are substantial differences in the within-pair similarity between MZ and DZ pairs, this is strong evidence that genes are responsible for the trait being measured. If that trait is the tendency towards development of a disease like Alzheimer's disease, then there will be differences in the proportions of twin pairs in which both members have the disease (concordant pairs) as opposed to those in which only one is affected (discordant pairs). Particularly when the population rates of a disease are known (i.e. the chance that another individual chosen at random will have the disease), one may apply statistical techniques to estimate the degree to which the predisposition to the disease is inherited, as well as the degree to which shared environmental influences contribute to a general tendency toward disease concordance in both types of twins. Thus, twin-researchers can estimate the relative contributions of genes, shared environmental influences, and other unique environmental influences (the residual after the first two are considered). This technique can provide important information that can guide the search for predisposing genes (when their influence is strong) and for environmental risk factors.

Four published twin studies of Alzheimer's disease all point to an important role for genes in determining susceptibility to Alzheimer's disease. One study, in relatively young men, suggested that the influence of genes was relatively modest (accounting for about one third of the population's variation in risk). One must remember, however, that the relative influences of genes and environmental factors might not remain constant as people age: genes typically predispose to the development of Alzheimer's disease in late old age, while environmental factors may increase the risk at earlier ages. Thus, we need to await the results of follow-up studies in the above cohort before concluding that its results are at any appreciable variance with other findings. The other studies, all conducted in older cohorts, suggest that genes account for 50–75% of the population's variation in risk of Alzheimer's disease.

What might these genes be? It is certain that, unlike the mutations at APP or the presenilins, they are not potent enough to assure the development of Alzheimer's disease in virtually all carriers; i.e. they are not *sufficient* to provoke the phenotype. It is less clear whether one gene, or one of several genes, may be *necessary* for development of the Alzheimer's disease phenotype. If so, then presumably some proportion of the population would lack the required gene or genes, and would not be susceptible to Alzheimer's disease. For the remainder, it is likely that several genes can modify an individual's risk of Alzheimer's disease, primarily by altering the age at which one is predisposed to develop the disease. The best known of these is *APOE*, the polymorphic genetic locus for the cholesterol transport protein, apolipoprotein E.

Apolipoprotein E (apoE) is unique among the family of lipoprotein fat transporters in its importance for brain development and repair. It is produced in the brain, which is second only to the liver in the amount of apoE produced. The protein product exists in three common isoforms: apoE2, apoE3 and apoE4. These variants are encoded by three different alleles (normal variations) in the *APOE* gene. The *APOE* system is similar to the well-known ABO family of blood groups. The alleles at *APOE* are called *APOE* ε2, ε3 and ε4. As in the ABO system, each person inherits one of these alleles from each parent. Thus, there are six possible genotypes (ε2/ε2, ε2/ε3, ε2/ε4, ε3/ε3, ε3/ε4 and ε4/ε4). These occur in frequencies that are predicted by the frequency of the three alleles. The ε2 allele is relatively rare; ε4 is somewhat more common; but ε3 is found on almost 78% of all chromosomes (Table 7.1).

The *APOE* system is the strongest known genetic determinant of susceptibility to late-onset Alzheimer's disease, but it is important to

TABLE 7.1

The *APOE* system and risk for Alzheimer's disease

Allele	Frequency (%)	Genotype	Frequency (%)	Implications for Alzheimer's disease
ε2	7	ε2/ε2	0.5	Not known
ε3	78	ε2/ε3	11	Probably later onset, reduced risk
ε4	15	ε2/ε4	2.0	Probably comparable to ε3/ε3
		ε3/ε3	61	Reference standard for this table
		ε3/ε4	23.5	Earlier onset, about threefold increased risk compared with ε3/ε3
		ε4/ε4	2.0	Much earlier onset; risk vs ε3/ε3 increased many-fold, depending on age

note that many people with even the risky ε4/ε4 genotype will not develop the disease even if they live to be 100. In animal models, too, *APOE* genotype predicts response to brain injury. Possession of the ε4 allele has been associated with less efficient acquisition of exploratory behaviors in young mice. There is also evidence from similar studies that the richness of synaptic development and dendritic outgrowth is reduced in transgenic mice with ε4. Finally, inheritance of an ε4 allele has been associated with slower recovery of mental ability after head injury.

The proportion of the total genetic influence mediated by *APOE* remains controversial. Most studies suggest that the relative risk with the ε4/ε4 genotype (compared with the common ε3/ε3 type) is between 12 and 20, while that with the ε3/ε4 genotype is between 2 and 4. Since about 2% of individuals bear the former and 24% the latter genotype, one may calculate population attributable risk for these genotypes (and, thus, for the ε4 allele altogether). Approached this way, it seems that ε4 may account for 50% of population variation in the risk of Alzheimer's disease. It is worth noting, however, that this estimate declines substantially after age 80 when Alzheimer's disease is most common.

There are numerous candidate genes that might explain the remaining genetic risk of Alzheimer's disease. Because these are all almost certainly weaker than *APOE*, they will be harder to detect. Correspondingly, larger and more powerful experiments will be required to show their effect. Smaller, underpowered experiments will predictably produce variable results – exactly what has been seen to date. More powerful family-based association methods or sib-pair linkage methods using high-resolution genome mapping techniques may offer the solution to this conundrum.

As a final caveat, we note that, particularly where relatively weak genes are concerned, inheritance does not equal fate. The twin studies suggest that about one third of the population's variation in Alzheimer's disease risk is environmental in origin. In Chapter 6, some of the environmental factors that may underlie this finding are discussed, several of which may suggest new roads to the prevention of Alzheimer's disease.

The 'free-radical hypothesis' of Alzheimer's disease

The association between Alzheimer's disease and aging has suggested that biological hypotheses to explain aging may prove relevant to understanding other causes of Alzheimer's disease. The major theories of aging include the 'free-radical hypothesis'. This idea would remain of interest only to Alzheimer researchers were it not for the repeated observation that individuals who take non-steroidal anti-inflammatory drugs (NSAIDs) have lower rates of dementia and mental impairment in late life. The following section explains what is happening when brain cells die in Alzheimer's disease and why NSAIDs might help prevent dementia.

Figure 7.3 shows how β-amyloid can be released from APP and bind to a large cell-surface molecule called the receptor for advanced glycation endproducts (RAGE). Interaction between β-amyloid and the walls of cerebral blood vessels probably causes oxidant stress. This

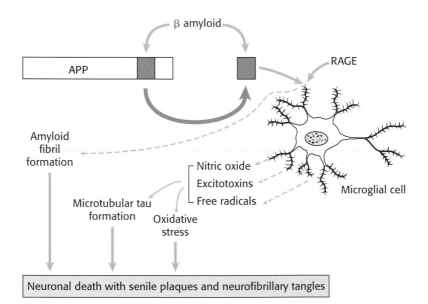

Figure 7.3 Release of β-amyloid from APP to bind at the receptor for advanced glycation endproducts (RAGE) leads to amyloid fibril formation, oxidative stress, then neuronal death with senile plaques and neurofibrillary tangles.

disturbs cellular function, damages intracellular proteins and causes cell death. In addition to their neurotoxic effects, β-amyloid fibrils stimulate microglia to produce neurotoxins (including reactive oxygen species, ROS). In turn, these trigger a cascade of toxic events central to the neurodegenerative process in Alzheimer's disease. Beta-amyloid fibrils and microglia probably interact through the scavenger receptor, which probably stimulates microglia to accumulate around β-amyloid deposits and so accounts for their proliferation in and around amyloid plaques.

The likely involvement of free-radical formation in this process is interesting but not compelling. Oxidative damage to neurons in Alzheimer's disease is as likely to be a consequence of neuronal damage as a cause of it. However, oxidative stress triggered by the deposition of β-amyloid fibrils could contribute significantly to worsening of neuronal injury. The location within the pathological segments of chromosome 21 of the gene coding for the enzyme superoxide dismutase, SOD-1, prompted a 'free-radical hypothesis' to account for Alzheimer's disease in Down's syndrome. Cultured neurons obtained from Down's syndrome fetuses generate increased amounts of ROS, presumably leading to neuronal death by apoptosis. This may account for abnormal brain development in Down's syndrome and, potentially, to the early onset of Alzheimer's disease in Down's syndrome.

The role of β-amyloid in the induction of brain cell death through stimulation of microglial activity, with the production of ROS, can be linked to the presence in neuritic plaques of cytokines which are released by cells when they are damaged, for example after a stroke, and orchestrate the inflammatory response. The 'amyloid toxicity hypothesis of Alzheimer's disease' and the 'free-radical theory of aging' are not mutually incompatible, and separately they can account for much Alzheimer-type degeneration in neurons. There is also some scope for interaction between the two processes. This possible interaction is supported by reports of the induction by β-amyloid of free-radical formation in blood vessels. β-amyloid can also activate neuronal membrane oxidation and so generate free radicals. Taken together these observations suggest that future studies will continue to support the neurotoxic effects of β-amyloid and may point to therapeutic strategies, such as vitamin E supplements in diet, which seek to preserve cerebrovascular endothelium and also reduce the neurotoxic effects of β-amyloid.

Tau protein, neurofibrillary tangles and Alzheimer's disease

The neuropathology of Alzheimer's disease includes the formation of neurofibrillary tangles (NFTs) in the limbic system and linked cortical sites. These become progressively more affected as the disease progresses. The nature and extent of the distribution of NFTs has been extensively studied and shows a close correlation with the degree of dementia. The molecular pathology of Alzheimer's disease is therefore more complex than would be suggested by successful navigation of the 'amyloid toxicity hypothesis'. The NFT contains paired helical filaments (PHFs) that are composed of tau protein present in an abnormally phosphorylated state. Tau is a member of a class of microtubule-associated proteins (MAPs) present throughout nervous tissue. At least six different types of MAP are present in adult brain, each of which is derived by differential processing of a single gene product. All six adult brain MAP types are hyperphosphorylated in Alzheimer's disease. In health, tau proteins (together with tubulin) promote polymerization of microtubules. When tau is hyperphosphorylated, such polymerization does not occur and tau subsequently forms PHFs that are the characteristic NFT lesions of Alzheimer's disease.

NFTs have proven very difficult to study, largely because of their relative insolubility. This feature also allows the NFT to survive after the death of a neuron and gives rise to the term 'tombstone' or 'ghost tangles'. Early research on the molecular pathology of Alzheimer's disease focused on the senile plaques, and it is only in the past few years that substantial progress has been made in understanding the molecular composition of NFTs. The progressive deposition of NFTs in cortical brain areas is known to follow a consistent pattern. This close relationship between pathological change and the stages of clinical dementia, together with the evidence that the formation of NFTs provides a better distinction between healthy aging and Alzheimer's disease than does the presence of senile plaques, has suggested to some researchers that the hyperphosphorylation of tau protein is the key step in the initiation of other molecular pathological events which produce the characteristic neuropathological changes of Alzheimer's disease. The molecular mechanisms involved that are currently being elucidated may provide a therapeutic target for novel drugs in the prevention of Alzheimer's disease.

Hypotheses on the causes of Alzheimer's disease – Key points

Genetics
- Genetic factors are relevant to all forms of Alzheimer's disease irrespective of age at onset or family history
- In rare, familial forms of early-onset dementia, faulty genes are involved in about 19% of cases. These code for a cellular adhesion molecule (amyloid precursor protein, APP) or for molecules involved in APP processing (presenilins).
- Population studies indicate that a substantial part – perhaps around 50–75% – of the risk of late-onset Alzheimer's disease is influenced by genetic factors
- Many genetic risk factors are unidentified. Polymorphisms in the *APOE* gene that encodes the lipid transport protein apolipoprotein E may determine timing of the onset of Alzheimer's disease but do not directly cause it.

Selective neuronal death
- Neuronal death in Alzheimer's disease is associated with amyloid production, stimulation of oxygen free-radical formation and hyperphosphorylation of the microtubule-associated protein tau.
- Selective hippocampal damage may be caused or aggravated by the neurotoxic actions of cortisol.

Key references

Albert MS, Jones K, Savage CR et al. Predictors of cognitive change in older persons: MacArthur studies of successful aging. *Psychol Aging* 1995;10:578–89.

Christensen H, Korten AE, Jorm AF et al. Education and decline in cognitive performance: compensatory but not protective. *Int J Geriatr Psychiatry* 1997;12:323–30.

Corder EH, Saunders AM, Strittmatter WJ et al. Gene dose of apolipoprotein E type 4 allele and the risk of Alzheimer's disease in late onset families. *Science* 1993;261:921–3.

David II JN, Chisholm JC. The 'amyloid cascade hypothesis' of AD: decoy or real McCoy? *Trends Neurosci* 1997;20:558–9.

De Strooper B, Saftig P, Craessaerts K et al. Deficiency of presenilin-1 inhibits the normal cleavage of amyloid precursor protein. *Nature* 1998;391:387–90.

Farrer LA, Cupples LA, van Duijn CM et al. Apolipoprotein E genotype in patients with Alzheimer's disease: implications for the risk of dementia among relatives. *Ann Neurol* 1995;38:797–808.

Goedert M. Tau protein and the neurofibrillary pathology of Alzheimer's disease. *Trends Neurosci* 1993;16:460–5.

Harman D. A theory based on free radical and radiation chemistry. *J Gerontol* 1956;11:298–300.

Mattson MP. Modification of ion homeostasis by lipid peroxidation: roles in neuronal degeneration and adaptive plasticity. *Trends Neurosci* 1998;21:53–7.

McClearn GE, Johansson B, Berg S et al. Substantial genetic influence on cognitive abilities in twins 80 or more years old. *Science* 1997;276:1560–3.

Poirier J. Apolipoprotein E in animal models of CNS injury and in Alzheimer's disease. *Trends Neurosci* 1994;17:525–30.

Roth GS, Joseph JA, Mason RP. Membrane alterations as causes of impaired signal transduction in Alzheimer's disease and aging. *Trends Neurosci* 1995;18:203–6.

Whalley LJ, Starr JM, Athawes R et al. Childhood mental ability and dementia. *Neurology* 2000;55:1455–9.

Caring for dementia patients

Family physicians are often the first point of contact between a suspected dementia patient and health services. Sophisticated investigations are occasionally needed, but most physicians should be able to exclude any physical disease that could account for the presentation. The MMSE forms a cornerstone for the clinical evaluation of dementia. It provides a useful measure of the nature and extent of cognitive deficits and is often a vital baseline against which any subsequent change, particularly a response to antidementia drugs, can be measured.

Early in the course of dementia assessment it is useful to establish with carers and sometimes with patients the possible causes that might account for the presentation. Many patients are aware of the differential diagnosis, and awkward questions are commonplace. Members of the clinical team need to consider how fully to answer these questions, whether or not to offer a precise diagnosis and how guardedly or otherwise to frame a prognosis. Presently, it is not uncommon to give a patient with early dementia good advice to help plan the next few years, and perhaps to influence treatment. Carers should routinely be made fully aware of likely diagnoses and the implications for future personal safety and independence.

In addition to diagnostic procedures, good clinical practice includes the assessment at home of continuing abilities to perform domestic chores and to drive a car, and an estimation of risk of self-harm because of failing cognitive ability. Figure 8.1 shows the types of decision made by a dementia care team. Usually, a patient and carer accept advice when car driving has become unsafe, possibly tempered with comment that driving insurance is often invalid in the presence of the problems caused by dementia.

It is also good practice to include in a management plan a date for formal diagnostic review, usually 6 months after presentation but maybe up to a year later. This follow-up visit can be very helpful for

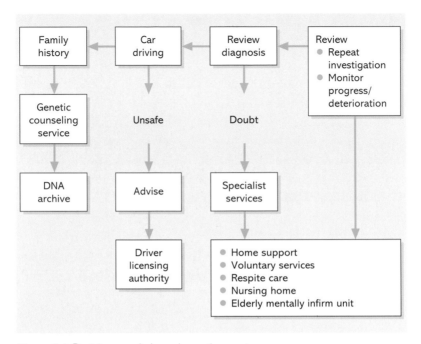

Figure 8.1 Decisions made by a dementia care team.

carers, particularly if no active treatment plan was put in place when diagnostic assessment was first completed. Memories of medical recommendation fade with time even when fully understood. Occasionally, the course of an apparent dementia will be atypical and suggest other diagnoses. This is particularly important when initial presentation was confounded by sedative drug use, a confusional state or exacerbation of systemic illness. Medical review also provides an opportunity for evaluation of the quality of care received by a dementia patient. Sometimes, a doctor or nurse is the only independent person able to do this on behalf of the patient. It is sometimes necessary to draw attention to the exploitation or even physical abuse of a dementia sufferer, and a diagnostic review is a good opportunity to make relevant observations.

Decisions about brain imaging, disclosure of diagnosis, unsafe car driving, genetic counseling, the management of behavioral complications of dementia, and the introduction of antidementia drugs, such as galantamine, rivastigmine and donepezil, are either deferred to secondary care or form part of a separate sequence of decisions (see Figure 8.1). Likewise, decisions are made about procedures to monitor care and response to drugs.

Nutritional assessment

Assessment of nutritional status is a key component of the examination of health in the elderly. Nutrition and lifestyle changes may increase the risk of loss of tissue function, and of diseases such as atherosclerosis and osteoporosis. Although total calorie requirements are lower in the elderly (around 1800–2100 kcal/day in men and about 400 kcal lower in women), there is widespread evidence that old people typically eat 10% less than this. Food frequency estimates based on usual dietary habits are notoriously unreliable in cognitively impaired subjects. There is also good evidence that old people receiving community care services are undernourished, and the same is often true of old people in residential care. Low body weight (detected as body mass index, BMI, below 20) and progressive weight loss are readily detected. Careful enquiry sometimes reveals low calorific intake, protein and antioxidant vitamins, vitamin B_{12} and folate. Demented patients are at high risk of malnutrition both at home and in residential care. When patients are poorly nourished, steps should be taken routinely to improve diet and to measure response to that intervention. Recommended daily dietary allowances for old people can be used to optimize nutrition. This is particularly important when poor diet and poverty coexist. When total food consumption is low, intake of essential vitamins can be quickly marginalized in old people. The use of vitamin supplements and additional fish oils is commonplace among health-conscious old people. There is some preliminary evidence (mostly from prospective observational studies) that dietary supplements promote retention of cognitive function in late life, and one randomized controlled trial suggests that supplementation with supraphysiological doses of α-tocopherol (vitamin E) will delay time to obligatory residential care in late-onset Alzheimer's disease.

Epidemiological studies confirm the importance of a good balanced diet to the maintenance of health in old age. The discovery that homocysteine is a risk factor for dementia lends weight to the nutritional advice that currently too little attention is paid to the promotion of adequate folate and vitamin B_{12} intake. The dangers of neuronal damage being caused by unopposed effects of folate are too slight to cause concerns about the addition of folate to cereals and other foodstuffs. There is also some longitudinal observational evidence that diets rich in fish oils (ω–3 fatty acids) with adequate antioxidants have brain protective benefits. Where the consumption of fish oils forms a significant part of the diet compared with vegetable oils (ω–6 fatty acids), there are data to suggest a lower incidence of dementia.

Behavioral problems

The management of behavioral problems in dementia is based on sound and consistent nursing and prescribing practice. Whenever possible, those involved in dementia care should be fully aware of local procedures. In nursing homes and dementia care units these procedures should be written down and subject to regular review. When an unwanted behavior is detected, carers should be encouraged to look for 'triggers' in the patient's circumstances that may be linked to onset or offset. These may include physiological sensations like the need to micturate. Simple reassurance often helps allay the fears of desertion or harm prompted by anxiety or uncertainty. Unfortunately for many carers, such reassurance may lead to intense feelings of dependency on the part of the sufferer, who may seek the near-continuous comforting presence of the carer. In such circumstances, skilled support may be necessary to afford the carer some respite. Table 8.1 shows non-drug interventions in behavioral problems in dementia.

When psychological and educational strategies fail, medication should be considered. The introduction of drugs must be balanced against their possible adverse effects. For sedative drugs, these effects include an apparent worsening of dementia, falls, cumulative toxicity, tolerance and withdrawal phenomena and the induction of extrapyramidal side-effects. The last are very troubling for dementia patients because their distress can sometimes be ignored when language is impaired and effects like akathisia or drooling are wrongly attributed to dementia and not the medication.

TABLE 8.1

Non-drug interventions in behavioral problems in dementia

- Reality orientation

  Accurate information about person and surroundings
- Behavioral analysis

  Detailed analysis of behavior, content and triggers
- Occupational activities

  Positive stimulation, e.g. music therapy
- Environmental modifications

  Changes in care routines, orientation cues
- Sensory stimulation

  Touch/massage, aromatherapy, bright light
- Education

  Carer-focused, social support measures

When drugs are used, attention should be paid to the patient's understanding and consent to treatment, drug choice, dose and duration. Subterfuge, coercion or physical restraint should not be used to administer a drug to a demented patient unless approved by a properly constituted authority that is legally permitted to grant such approval. It is better to avoid sedative drugs, including benzodiazepines, whenever possible. If there is no alternative, these drugs should be used in the lowest effective dose and withdrawn within 1 month. Generally, older demented patients are more sensitive to the ill-effects of drugs used to control behavioral symptoms or signs. It is good practice to start at the lowest dose and increase gradually at intervals of at least five times the half-life of the selected drug. Drug prescribing guidelines whenever possible should be agreed in residential facilities. A useful rule is 'start low, go slow'. Medical review of prescribing should include steps to detect inadvertent or deliberate administration to the patient of drugs intended for another (perhaps a carer or fellow resident). Table 8.2 lists drugs commonly used to treat behavioral symptoms in dementia. As a general rule, drugs should be used only for serious

TABLE 8.2

Drugs used to treat behavioral problems in dementia

Neuroleptics	Non-neuroleptics
• Haloperidol	• Chlormethiazole
• Chlorpromazine	• Benzodiazepines
• Olanzapine	• Antidepressants
• Risperidone	• Anticonvulsants
	• Lithium

problems, the treatment of delusions and hallucinations, risk of injury to self or others, or in the presence of severe and persistent distress. Neuroleptic drugs are used frequently, but there is little evidence to support this practice. Doses determined in trials to treat schizophrenia do not reliably guide prescribing in demented old people. In addition to neuroleptic drugs and anticonvulsants (for aggression), antidepressants are often used, though again there is little formal evidence to support their use in dementia.

Acetylcholinesterase inhibitors

The cholinergic system is important to learning and memory. Surgical lesions of cholinergic fibers in animal studies, pharmacological studies of anticholinergic agents, and neurochemical studies in aging and Alzheimer's disease all support the idea that the functions of intact cholinergic neurons are essential to learning and memory. Between 1972 and 1980, such studies laid the basis for almost two decades of therapeutic research on the cholinergic system in Alzheimer's disease. At first, it appeared that reduced cholinergic function was specific for Alzheimer's disease and not found in other types of dementia. Cross-diagnostic studies with adequate control samples found that in postmortem brain tissues, levels of enzymes associated with the synthesis (choline acetyl transferase, ChAT) and degradation (acetylcholinesterase, AChE) were reduced in Alzheimer's disease and also, but to a lesser extent, in aging in the absence of dementia, alcoholic dementia, dementia associated with Parkinson's disease and in some instances of vascular dementia. The conclusion that the cholinergic deficit was specific to Alzheimer's disease was soon abandoned.

Over the past 30 years, many attempts have been made to enhance cholinergic function in Alzheimer's disease. Compounds that contained precursors of acetylcholine or mimicked its actions in the brain were tested but none proved successful. However, acetylcholinesterase inhibitors now provide a sound foundation to the drug management of dementia. Three drugs are currently available in most countries:

- donepezil
- rivastigmine
- galantamine.

Their pharmacological profiles are broadly similar but there are several important differences in pharmocokinetic properties and information on safety and benefits in routine clinical practice.

It is useful to summarize the benefits of the acetylcholinesterase inhibitors licensed for use in Alzheimer's disease. The case was convincingly made by manufacturers and accepted by licensing authorities that this group of drugs is of great potential benefit to the majority of individuals with mild-to-moderate Alzheimer's disease. The economic case for the use of this class of drugs is not based simply on Alzheimer's disease. It is closely linked to the problem of disability in old people. Current cognitive function is a major determinant of disability in old age – so much so that around 40% of disabled people aged 65 years and over are cognitively impaired. About 50% of people in institutional care are cognitively impaired, and this is now the main reason for such care. Dementia also contributes to hospitalization and disability in other ways. For example, a reduction of dementia prevalence of 1–2% would reduce the number of hip fractures in the UK by 20 000 per year.

The institutionalization of dementia sufferers varies widely between localities. In general, dementia patients are about four times more likely to move into institutional care when compared with an age-matched population. Around 30% of memory clinic patients are reported to move into residential care within a year of first attending the clinic.

These moves are explained by disease progression. Activities of Daily Living (ADL) scores are valid measures of disease progression.

These acetylcholinesterase inhibitors possess the potential to reduce disability and institutionalization rates. One early study of patients receiving tacrine showed that long-term doses greater than 80 mg/day reduced the likelihood of admission to a nursing home compared with those on lower doses or who had stopped the drug. Analysis of the complex tasks component of an ADL measure collected during a double-blind, randomized controlled trial of donepezil showed active treatment groups improved when compared with placebo, with statistical significance for the 10 mg/day donepezil dose. Subjects who tolerated a daily dose of 6 mg or more of rivastigmine had unchanged personal ADL scores over 6 months, compared with a significant decline for those receiving either less than 6 mg or placebo.

It is sometimes suggested that acetylcholinesterase inhibitors prolong the overall time from disease onset to death and this has been used to argue against their use. Effects of treatment on institutionalization can be estimated. Using rivastigmine data, doses of at least 6 mg daily reduce institutionalization by 8–14% per year. This compares with the accepted effect of stroke unit care of a 1.5% absolute reduction. There have now been 13 randomized placebo-controlled trials of the three acetylcholinesterase inhibitors under consideration (4 with donepezil, 4 with rivastigmine and 5 with galantamine). Most studies were designed to demonstrate superiority of the target drug over placebo in terms of cognitive function and a clinician's impression-of-change measure. The consensus view is that the benefit of this class of drugs approximates to an average delay of over 6 months when compared with placebo-treated patients. There is up to a 50% prevalence of a 4 point or greater improvement over placebo on the ADAS-cog, a scale rating cognitive change. About 50% of responders show an effect size of 7 or more points on the ADAS-cog. Many studies also report ADL scores and show benefits consistent with improved cognitive scores. ADL benefits are somewhat smaller but seem likely to be relevant to reduced disability and the delay of institutionalization.

In general, acetylcholinesterase inhibitors are well tolerated, with donepezil perhaps better tolerated than others. The most common adverse reactions relate to cholinergic effects on the gastrointestinal tract (nausea, vomiting and diarrhea) with an excess of actively treated patient withdrawals over placebo of approximately 5%.

Data from Canada indicate that institutionalization is responsible for the largest part of dementia costs. Economic predictions suggest that use of donepezil for mild-to-moderate Alzheimer's disease reduces 5-year costs and lessens the time spent in the severe phase of Alzheimer's disease when compared with the alternative of usual care. In US patients with Alzheimer's disease who were being cared for at home at the start of a 6-month study period, treatment with donepezil did not increase overall direct medical costs. To achieve in one patient an improvement of 4 points on the ADAS-cog in excess of the response that would be expected by chance, between four and six patients would need to be treated with donepezil 10 mg once daily for 6 months.

Routine clinical experience in the 'real world' outside the clinical trial setting where all patients receive active drug, indicates that about one half of patients show some cognitive improvement and a minority improve quite markedly. The typical response in Alzheimer's disease to an acetylcholinesterase inhibitor is subtle but with identifiable improvement within 12 weeks in attentiveness, apathy, conversational language and ADL, sufficient to make some difference to those caring for the patient. In addition, patients with behavioral problems often show the most clinically significant benefit as assessed by carers and formal assessments such as the Neuropsychiatric Inventory (NPI) and its carer distress scale. The Southampton Memory Clinic found that 49% of patients showed improvement from baseline and 37% showed an improvement of 4 points or greater on the NPI. Therefore it is safe to draw the following conclusions for acetylcholinesterase inhibitors.

- There are clear benefits of treatment in terms of delay in cognitive decline and ADL and amelioration of neuropsychiatric symptoms.
- The less well-documented but clinically very important effects such as the neuropsychiatric benefit and the benefit to carers' wellbeing are of great value in clinical practice.
- Reduction in institutionalization rates following treatment are greater than those seen following stroke unit care.

- The economic case remains not proven, but drug costs are likely to be outweighed by delayed institutionalization costs in the absence of an effect on survival.

Specific acetylcholinesterase inhibitors are as follows.

Tacrine (tetrahydroaminoacridine) was the first drug to be registered, and there are at least 21 published trials. These established efficacy in mild-to-moderate Alzheimer's disease in both cognitive and behavioral symptoms. Withdrawal-from-treatment rates are much higher for tacrine than for other acetylcholinesterase inhibitors. Most withdrawals are tacrine-related, of which one third are caused by raised liver enzymes and two thirds by cholinergic side-effects. The drug is unavailable in the UK but continues to be used widely in many countries. When donepezil and/or rivastigmine are also available, tacrine use quickly declines, largely because it needs to be taken four times daily, compared with once daily for donepezil and twice daily for rivastigmine.

Donepezil (Aricept) is a reversible acetylcholinesterase inhibitor highly selective for acetylcholinesterase and much less so for butyrylcholinesterase. Half-life is around 3 days, peak plasma concentration is attained within 3–4 hours and steady-state plasma concentrations within 15 days (equivalent to five half-lives of the drug). There are substantial data, including results from two 1-year placebo-controlled studies, to support moderate but consistent benefits of this drug in Alzheimer's disease.

Rivastigmine (Exelon) is an acetylcholinesterase inhibitor with specific selectivity for brain acetylcholinesterase. The half-life of rivastigmine is uncertain; it is quickly metabolized and needs to be taken twice daily. The drug has the lowest risk of drug interactions in its class – it is not metabolized by hepatic microsomal (cytochrome P450) enzymes – but in routine clinical practice there seems to be little difference between donepezil and rivastigmine in terms of efficacy or adverse events. Some physicians find donepezil is better tolerated than rivastigmine.

Galantamine (galanthamine) differs from donepezil and rivastigmine because it also modifies nicotinic cholinergic receptors.

This may account for pharmacological differences, but it is not associated with clinical advantage.

Side-effects of acetylcholinesterase inhibitors. This class of drugs shares common side-effects on the gastrointestinal system (nausea, vomiting) some dizziness, anorexia and transient confusion. For all three drugs, these effects are brief and usually subside within 2 weeks. Titration of drug dose is more necessary with rivastigmine than donepezil, but this is rarely a problem. Because of effects on appetite, weight should be monitored throughout treatment. Absolute contraindications to their use are few, but include sick sinus and other conduction defects.

Practical aspects of acetylcholinesterase inhibitor use. Therapy should be initiated once the Alzheimer's disease diagnosis is likely and there are no contraindications. Advanced age is not a contraindication. It is usual to withdraw concomitant medication about 3 weeks before initiation of therapy. An ECG is not routinely necessary but should be performed if there are irregularities in pulse. At baseline, clinical chemistry, including liver enzymes, should be recorded and reviewed at 3 months and 1 year. Evidence of efficacy is an important determinant of continuation therapy and should be sought using a standardized scale; though not designed for the purpose, many clinicians find the total MMSE score to be an adequate guide to changes in disease severity. Decisions to withdraw drug in the face of lack of efficacy, usually after 12–18 months, can be supported by an MMSE decline of more than 5 points in the face of adequate acetylcholinesterase inhibitor dose over a year of treatment.

Memantine

Memantine is a derivative of the antiviral drug amantidine which was unexpectedly found to reduce the symptoms of Parkinson's disease. Like amantidine, memantine is a weak promoter of dopamine release but is a much stronger antagonist of a receptor involved in cell death through a mechanism called 'excitotoxicity'. These receptors are normally activated by the amino acid L-glutamate which is the major excitatory transmitter in the brain. Receptors stimulated by glutamate are present in several forms; one of which is selectively stimulated by the amino acid analog N-methyl-D-aspartate (NMDA) and is known as the NMDA receptor. Memantine is a specific antagonist of the NMDA receptor. When stimulated, NMDA receptors allow calcium to enter the neuron and trigger biochemical changes that underpin modifications of synaptic function involved in memory and learning. The activity of large cortical pyramidal neurons represents a delicate balance between excitatory (glutamate) and inhibitory (GABA) inputs. Excessive and prolonged stimulation of NMDA receptors disrupts this balance and is highly toxic to neurons (glutamate excitotoxicity). When this stimulation causes neurons to be overloaded with calcium, many calcium-dependent enzymes (proteases) are over-activated and there is excess generation of free radicals. This type of 'glutamate excitotoxicity' is probably involved in cell death after stroke, in poorly controlled epilepsy and in some age-related neurodegenerative diseases like Huntington's disease and Alzheimer's disease.

Memantine is of modest value in the treatment of Parkinson's disease, and this has encouraged its use in the treatment of other age-related neurodegenerative conditions since about 1990. Evidence from current randomized clinical trials of memantine in Alzheimer's disease is awaited but two relevant studies are available. In one Swedish study, 82 patients with severe dementia (MMSE scores < 10 points) received memantine 10 mg per day, while 84 received placebo. Dementia diagnoses comprised both Alzheimer's disease and vascular dementia but may also have included mixed types. After 12 weeks, care needs were slightly but significantly less with memantine than with placebo. In the second study, French patients with vascular dementia (MMSE scores 12–20) were randomly assigned to memantine 20 mg daily or placebo. After 28 weeks, scores on ADAS-cog showed significant advantages of memantine over placebo. At present it is too early to assess the possible role of memantine in the treatment of Alzheimer's disease. Benefits of memantine therapy seem likely in the treatment of vascular dementia. Cerebrovascular pathology is commonplace in late-onset Alzheimer's disease and may be intimately involved in the pathogenesis of amyloid formation.

Encouraging results were reported in conference proceedings in 2002 from at least one adequately sized trial in patients with severe Alzheimer's disease. Those treated with memantine showed negligible progression of their symptom severity over a year of observation, whereas those treated with placebo declined predictably.

Principles of care and current treatment – Key points

- Dementia care is best provided by a dementia team with a range of skills to investigate, treat and support patients and carers.
- Nutritional status is a key part of dementia assessment; dementia signs and symptoms may improve when nutrition is optimized.
- Drug treatments of behavioral symptoms should only be used after non-drug interventions have been tried. When used, medication should be initiated at low doses and be increased slowly if necessary ('Start low, go slow').
- For those with mild-to-moderate dementia in whom the presence of Alzheimer-type pathology seems likely, acetylcholinesterase inhibitor treatment should be considered, irrespective of age.

Key references

Coons DH. *Specialized Dementia Care Units*. Baltimore: Johns Hopkins University Press, 1991.

Eccles M, Clarke J, Livingstone M et al. North of England evidence based guidelines development project: guideline for primary care management of dementia. *BMJ* 1998;317:802–8.

Orogozo JM, Rigaud AS, Stoffler A et al. Efficacy and safety of memantine in patients with mild to moderate vascular dementia – a randomised placebo-controlled trial (MMM300). *Stroke* 2002;33: 1834–9.

Rabins PV, Lyketsos CG, Steele CD. *Practical Dementia Care*. Oxford: Oxford University Press, 1999.

Rogers SL, Friedhoff LT. Long-term efficacy and safety of donepezil in the treatment of Alzheimer's disease: an interim analysis of the results of a US multicentre open label extension study. *Eur Neuropsychopharmacol* 1998;8:67–75.

Rosler M, Anand R, Cicin-Sain A et al. Efficacy and safety of rivastigmine in patients with Alzheimer's disease: international randomised controlled trial. *BMJ* 1999;318:633–8.

Starr JM, Whalley LJ, Deary IJ. The effects of antihypertensive treatment on cognitive function: results from the HOPE study. *J Am Geriatr Soc* 1996;44:411–15.

Winblatt B, Poritis N. Memantine in severe dementia: results of the M-9-BEST study (benefit and efficacy in severely demented patients during treatment with memantine). *Int J Ger Psychiat* 1999;14:135–46.

9 Future treatments

In the previous chapter we have described prescription treatments that may improve the cognitive performance of people with dementia. The model for the development of these drugs was the earlier finding that L-dopa treatment produced symptomatic improvement in Parkinson's disease. The most prominent neurochemical deficit in Alzheimer's disease is reduced availability of acetylcholine (ACh). Oral administration of metabolic precursors of ACh (like phosphatidyl choline or lecithin) has proven difficult because of unpleasant gastrointestinal side-effects, and because the treatment is a nutritionally undesirable saturated fat. The current drug treatments therefore attempt to increase availability of ACh by impeding its degradation after release into the synaptic space (see Chapter 1). The enzyme responsible for this degradation is acetylcholinesterase (AChE). All currently approved Alzheimer's disease treatments are inhibitors of AChE. Sadly, unlike L-dopa, which offers good benefit to the great majority of those with early-to-moderate stage Parkinson's disease, AChE inhibition appears to offer only relatively modest benefits in only a minority of Alzheimer's patients.

Just as L-dopa treatment does not reverse or attenuate the underlying course of Parkinson's disease, inhibition of AChE probably has little effect on the march of pathological changes that underlies the progression of Alzheimer's disease. An ideal treatment effect would be the inhibition of this chain of pathological events. Obviously, to produce such inhibition requires knowledge of the key events. At present, however, theories of Alzheimer's disease pathogenesis are only partially worked out and sometimes competing. Those who are persuaded that Aβ is the culprit would direct research efforts toward inhibition of amyloidogenesis. Others, convinced that the neurofibrillary tangle is the key Alzheimer's disease lesion, would look for ways to prevent the hyperphosphorylation of tau and related microtubule-associated proteins. While pharmaceutical companies are spending many millions of pounds pursuing these avenues, any resulting commercially available treatments are several years away from testing in clinical trials.

The potential public health importance of dementia prevention or slowing of disease onset was well illustrated by Ron Brookmeyer and his colleagues at Johns Hopkins University School of Medicine. Using available US incidence data and models to forecast the age and sex structure of the US population, they estimated the absolute numbers of Alzheimer cases prevented if effective measures to slow onset were introduced. Table 9.1 is adapted from their work and shows that even a modest slowing of 6 months will reduce the number of cases by 100 000 within 10 years of its introduction. A delay of 1 year is more dramatic, reducing the number of new cases by 200 000. From a UK perspective, these numbers translate into reductions of about 18 000 and 36 000 for 6 months and 1 year, respectively.

An expedient approach is to pursue empirical epidemiological findings, even when these are not fully explained by current theory. For example, the risk of Alzheimer's disease appears to be reduced among those who are long-term users of hormone replacement therapy, statins, NSAIDs, and possibly of histamine-H2-blockers, and of antioxidants

TABLE 9.1

Potential effects on the prevalence of Alzheimer's disease of interventions to delay onset of the disease in the US population after introduction as a public-health measure from 1998

Relative risk of intervention	Mean delay (years)	Alzheimer disease prevalence (million cases)	
		2007	2027
1.00	0	2.89	4.74
0.95	0.5	2.79	4.52
0.90	1.0	2.68	4.31
0.75	2.0	2.32	3.64
0.50	5.0	1.74	2.49

From Brookmeyer et al. *Am J Public Health* 1998;88:1337–42.

like vitamins E and C and perhaps red wine. A logical sequence of experimentation is required if these observations are eventually to yield medicines that can be used either to treat or prevent Alzheimer's disease. Particularly for the less well-established approaches, we need repetitions of existing observations using more rigorous study designs. Such designs must overcome a common difficulty in retrospective studies: determination of which drugs or vitamins have been used over the years. To some extent, this problem can be solved using prospective (incidence–cohort) designs, but the follow-up observation period in such studies is often lengthy. This makes for an extended period of investigation, and it also creates difficulty in learning which subjects (regardless of their original status as drug users or non-users) may have used the 'treatments' in the lengthy intervening interval.

However, even a perfect prospective observational study could not be considered conclusive, because its subjects would be 'self-assigned' into groups that use or do not use the drug under investigation. The self-assignment process (decision whether to use the drug of interest) can reflect attributes (health consciousness, general medical health, or even concern about memory difficulties) that may be related to the outcome, incident Alzheimer's disease. Thus, randomized controlled trials will be needed to test the most promising empirical candidates for prevention and treatment of Alzheimer's disease.

Since Alzheimer's disease appears to be a chronic disease with latent, prodromal and active symptomatic phases, there are three stages at which trials may be used to test the benefit of potential treatments:

- in the latent stage, to prevent progression to later phases in at-risk individuals (primary prevention)
- in the prodromal stage, to prevent progression of age-related cognitive decline or its march to dementia (secondary prevention)
- in established dementia, to prevent progression of symptoms (tertiary prevention).

In each stage, the aim will be to demonstrate prevention of disease progression rather than symptomatic improvement.

Primary prevention. There is considerable interest in the potential of hormone replacement therapy and NSAIDs for primary prevention of

Alzheimer's disease. Randomized controlled primary prevention trials of each are currently beginning. Because of their safety and ease of use, antioxidant vitamins and H2-blockers could be added on to these trials, perhaps using a factorial design. These studies are very expensive and will require at least 5 years to complete.

Secondary prevention in patients with minimal cognitive impairment. Several randomized trials are now underway to test whether administration of NSAIDs that selectively inhibit the Cox-2 isoform of cyclooxygenase can prevent progression of severity in age-related cognitive decline, or its eventual march to dementia. Data will probably be available in the next 2 years. There are no known ongoing trials of this type using conventional NSAIDs.

Tertiary prevention: attenuation of disease progression. One observational study and two small randomized trials have suggested that NSAIDs may slow the progression of fully symptomatic Alzheimer's dementia. The observational study considered the 1-year decline in cognitive test scores among 202 patients enrolled at a university Alzheimer's disease clinic. The patients were classified as NSAID users or non-users on admission to the clinic. The study suggested that NSAID users had a significantly lower rate of decline on several cognitive tests.

Even if the chronic disease model is correct, a treatment that is effective in one stage may not be effective in another. As the disease process progresses, there is a corresponding destruction of the integrity of the nervous system. There are well known phenomena of anterograde and retrograde degeneration that may result in the loss of healthy neurons that would not be otherwise attacked by the primary Alzheimer's disease process. Some have therefore argued that the pathogenesis of Alzheimer's disease may at some point become 'autocatalytic', implying the existence of a point at which amelioration or attenuation of the primary Alzheimer's disease lesioning process will have a reduced or absent effect on the continued progression of the disease. The implication is that treatments that are effective for prevention (particularly for primary prevention) may lose their effectiveness beyond a certain point in the progression of the Alzheimer's disease process. We therefore confront a dilemma: the treatment strategies that are most convenient and economical to test may have the lowest likelihood of success.

Indeed, this principle may explain the lack of success of several recent treatment trials with a potent anti-inflammatory drug, prednisone (prednisolone in the UK), with a selective Cox-2 inhibiting NSAID, and with estrogen-replacement therapy. An earlier trial with the antioxidant vitamin E and the anti-Parkinson's drug selegiline (also with powerful antioxidant potential) was more hopeful, but failed to demonstrate any change in the rate of decline in cognitive abilities in Alzheimer's disease. Given the urgent need for effective preventative strategies in Alzheimer's disease, the most promising interventions should be tested over the next decade at all stages of illness.

Future treatments – Key points

- Important developments are expected in drug treatments to prevent amyloid neurotoxicity.
- Homocysteine- and lipid-lowering strategies as well as anti-inflammatory and antioxidant interventions are currently under investigation for the prevention or slowing of dementia onset.

Key references

Gould E, Beylin A, Tanapat P et al. Learning enhances adult neurogenesis in the hippocampal formation. *Nat Neurosci* 1999;2:260–5.

Jick H, Zornberg GL, Jick SS et al. Statins and the risk of dementia. *Lancet* 2000;356:1627–31.

Lowenstein DH, Parent JM. Brain, heal thyself. *Science* 1999;283: 1126–7.

McKay R. Stem cells in the central nervous system. *Science* 1997;276: 66–71.

Rottkamp CA, Nunomura A, Hirai K et al. Will antioxidants fulfill their expectations for the treatment of Alzheimer disease? *Mech Ageing Dev* 2000;116:169–79.

Rozzini R, Ferrucci L, Losonczy K et al. Protective effect of chronic NSAID use on cognitive decline in older persons. *J Am Geriatr Soc* 1996;44:1025–9.

Scheffler B, Horn M, Blumcke I et al. Marrow-mindedness: a perspective on neuropoiesis. *Trends Neurosci* 1999;22:348–57.

Schmidt R, Fazekas F, Reinhart B et al. Estrogen replacement therapy in older women: a neuropsychological and brain MRI study. *J Am Geriatr Soc* 1996;44:1307–13.

Vaughan CJ, Delanty N. Neuroprotective properties of statins in cerebral ischaemia and stroke. *Stroke* 1999;30:1969–73.

Appendix: useful addresses

Alzheimer Europe
145 Route de Thionville
2611 Luxembourg
fax: +352 297972
www.alzheimer-europe.org

Alzheimer's Association
919 North Michigan Avenue,
Suite 1100, Chicago,
IL 60611-1676, USA
US toll-free phone: 800 272 3900
fax: +1 312 335 1110
www.alz.org

**Alzheimer's Disease Education
and Referral (ADEAR) Center**
PO Box 8250, Silver Spring,
MD 20907-8250, USA
US toll-free phone: 800 438 4380
www.alzheimers.org

Alzheimer's Disease International
45–46 Lower Marsh,
London SE1 7RG, UK
phone: +44 20 7620 3011
fax: +44 20 7401 7351
info@alz.co.uk
www.alz.co.uk

Alzheimer's Research Forum
www.alzforum.org

Alzheimer's Research Trust
Livanos House, Granhams Road,
Cambridge, CB2 5LQ, UK
phone: +44 1223 843899
fax: +44 1223 843325
enquiries@alzheimers-research.
org.uk
www.alzheimers-research.co.uk

Alzheimer's Society
Gordon House, 10 Greencoat
Place, London SW1P 1PH, UK
phone: +44 20 7306 0606
fax: +44 20 7306 0808
enquiries@alzheimers.org.uk
www.alzheimers.org.uk

Alzheimer Society of Canada
20 Eglinton Ave W, Ste 1200,
Toronto, ON M4R 1K8, Canada
phone: +1 416 488 8772
Canadian toll-free phone:
1 800 616 8816
fax: +1 416 488 3778
info@alzheimer.ca
www.alzheimer.ca

Dementia Research Group
The National Hospital for
Neurology and Neurosurgery,
Queens Square,
London WC1N 3BG, UK
phone: +44 20 7829 8773
fax: +44 870 132 0447
enquiries@dementia.ion.ucl.ac.uk
dementia.ion.ucl.ac.uk

Index